4.95

THE SELF AND AUTISM

THE LIBRARY OF ANALYTICAL PSYCHOLOGY
Volume 3

THE SELF AND AUTISM

MICHAEL FORDHAM

William Heinemann Medical Books Ltd
London

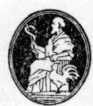

First published 1976

© The Society of Analytical Psychology Ltd, 1976

ISBN 0 433 30882 6

Text set in 11/12 pt. Monotype Baskerville, printed by letterpress, and bound in Great Britain at The Pitman Press, Bath

THE LIBRARY OF ANALYTICAL PSYCHOLOGY

Edited by

MICHAEL FORDHAM
ROSEMARY GORDON
JUDITH HUBBACK
KENNETH LAMBERT

Contents

Editorial introduction

This, the third volume in the Library of Analytical Psychology, is the first single-author volume to appear in this collection. It has seemed to us entirely appropriate that it should be devoted to the writings of Michael Fordham, for he has been especially instrumental in protecting Jung's theories from the congealing effect of idealization. Instead, by drawing on his own experience of children and the treatment of children he has extended and developed many of Jung's key concepts. There is, in particular, his study and clarification of Jung's concept of the self, of archetypes, of the process of individuation and especially his own contribution of the concepts of the 'original self' and of 'deintegration' of this original self.

In this book Michael Fordham offers the reader a glimpse into the 'workshop' of those thoughts, reflections and clinical work and data that have formed the matrix of his most seminal ideas.

His study and treatment of autistic children seem to have led him to an operational understanding of the psychic institution of the self, for in these children he encountered the self in its psychopathological state when the defences and resistances to its natural 'deintegrative' process are in fact excessive.

Being here primarily concerned with patients in the first half of life, Fordham has been fascinated by the interaction of the functions of the ego and the self. In consequence he has re-assessed such processes as the religious experience in childhood, symbol formation and, most importantly, the process of individuation. Jung had tended to consider individuation as a process that occurs mainly, perhaps only, in the second half of life. Fordham's work with children convinced him that this was too narrow a view of individuation, that its essential characteristics can already be discerned in early childhood and that indeed its very roots have to be sought there. He holds the view that individuation is closely related and relevant to the achievement of awareness of personal identity and unit status and that really, as Rosemary Gordon would put it, individuation without individualization cannot but be false and illusory. And since individualization is primarily a result of the functions of the ego, the whole process of individuation, even though it may in many cases gather momentum in the later years of life, must be firmly anchored in the early years of life.

The value of the work Fordham expounds in this particular book lies then, above all, in his discovery in infancy and early childhood of the roots of some of our deeply significant, deeply personal and culturally important experiences.

The book is divided into three parts. The first contains the theoretical reflections and conclusions. The second part deals with clinical practice. The third part is composed entirely of the detailed description of the autistic children whose material and treatment had originally inspired Michael Fordham to write this book.

As has become customary in the volumes of the Library of Analytical Psychology, references to Jung's writings are here also taken from the 'Collected Works', which is abbreviated 'Coll. wks.' followed by the volume number. Dates refer to the first publication in whatever language and not to the English translation.

The author acknowledges with gratitude the opportunity to draw on the case material he gathered while working at the London Child Guidance Clinic and at the Paddington Child Guidance Clinic, and for the stimulus and support he received there from his colleagues, in particular from the late Dr. William Moody and from Dr. R. D. Newton.

The author also gratefully acknowledges permission to quote from his previously published works:

The British Journal of Medical Psychology **33**, 1. (1960. 'Counter-transference.')

Harvest 9. (1963. 'Myths, archetypes and patterns of child-hood'.)

Heinemann (1973. In *Analytical psychology: a modern Science*.)

Hodder & Stoughton (1969. *Children as Individuals*.)

S. Karger AG. Basel (1964. 'The theory of archetypes' in 'Der Archetyp' ed. by Guggenbuhl-Craig) and (1965. 'The Self in Childhood' in Proceedings of the 6th International Congress for Psychotherapy.)

The Journal of Analytical Psychology **3**, 2. (1958. 'Individuation and ego development'.)

Nervous child **6,** 3. (1947. Integration, disintegration and early
ego development'.)

Routledge and Kegan Paul (1944. *The life of childhood*) (1952.
New Developments in analytical psychology.) ('Collected Works
by C. G. Jung'.)

Finally, special thanks are due to Diana Riviere and to John
Lucas for their professional help in preparing this volume also
for publication.

Preface

This volume is the culmination of my work on the self in childhood. Its contents are dominated throughout by the ideas of Jung, though it may seem to many that I have departed rather far from what he intended. The departures may be covered by the following statement: Jung is generally held to have thought that the problems of individuation and of self-realization were primarily those of later life and not of childhood, though there are also indications—as Jacobi maintained—that he thought they could be applied to the whole span of life. My own investigations have given importance to childhood as the time when the ground plan of individuation is laid down, and I regard this work as valuable, but I agree that a whole class of people display the features that Jung described, and that they clearly show a general feature of maturation in 'the second half of life'. There is no contradiction in saying that the self and individuation are important in childhood, adolescence and the 'first half of life' also.

There has, however, been a curious reaction to my views, mostly privately expressed. The ideas that emerge have been so peculiar that I should scarcely like to mention them were it not that they appear to be influential. It is claimed, quite correctly, that the characteristic feature of Jung's work was his emphasis on the spiritual and religious life of human beings (I may remark in passing that I have published a contribution to this aspect of his work in a volume called *The objective psyche*, which was not ill thought of by him) but there has arisen among some analytical psychologists an idea that drawing attention to infancy and childhood means the denigration of Jung's work, presumably because children, unlike Jung himself, do not have spiritual or religious conflicts. There seems, further, to be an idea that, as in some primitive communities where the word 'child' is equated with 'nothing', childhood is insignificant. Then some have considered it a positively wicked view to think that infants and children have bodies and even feed at the breast and develop fantasies about it; worse still, they have excretary organs and genitals that, like the breast, are centres of affective conflict that influence their lives as adult persons. It appears that Jungian children do not have any of these organs, or if they do they certainly do not have any significant conflicts or fantasies about them. Only Freudian children or Kleinian babies are afflicted with such troubles. So it is said that I am more of a 'Freudian' or a 'Kleinian' than a 'Jungian'!

It is, of course, true that I have studied the work of psychoanalysts—as Jung did too—and have learned a great deal from them, and that I feel myself particularly fortunate to have practised in London, where the relationship between the two schools has been active and productive, but I doubt very much whether either Freudians or Kleinians would accept me as one of 'them'. Surely, if analytical psychology is to be thought of as a science—as Jung vigorously maintained it was—the conflict between schools needs to be worked out in detail and not reflected by sectarian prejudice, which has no place in any real development or progress in knowledge. To clarify the conflict I have included special chapters on my relationship to psychoanalytic concepts such as the religious experiences of children.

The central feature of this volume remains Jung's concept of the self. This was always related to clinical investigations. His concept and his method are of the first importance and they have proved to be so when applied to childhood. Following Jung, I have kept every step in the development of my ideas closely related to analytic observations. The first part of what I have written here may seem to do violence to this proposition in that it is exclusively theoretical, but this is so only because the observations on which the theory is based have already been published in *New developments in analytical psychology*, which those interested may refer to. To gain a more comprehensive view of how I conceive a child's development as a whole, in relation to his family and the social setting in which that family lives, it will be necessary to refer to *Children as individuals*, published in 1969.

I did not previously put forward the concept of the self as a defence system designed to establish and maintain a child's individuality until I was able to discover this through my investigations into infantile autism, which I now present here in detail for the first time.

Analytical observations are inevitably dependent upon the practices that the investigator employs. It is not justifiable to present conclusions without giving some account, however inadequate, of the methods used to arrive at them. I have therefore included in this book three chapters in order to give some account of my practices and of the ideas and methods I use; here again further information will be found in my earlier publications, and I hope to publish more on the difficult subject of technique.

It would require a special volume to deal satisfactorily with a description of Jungian method, technique and practice because so little has been written on it by analytical psychologists; indeed, only one volume entirely devoted to it has ever been published—Volume Two in this Library: *Technique in Jungian analysis*.

PART I

CHAPTER ONE

The theory of the archetypes and the self*

Introduction

In 'The origins of the ego in childhood' I published some ideas on the ego in the first two years of life. My intention was to develop a thesis implied in Jung's formulations as follows: consciousness, of which the ego is the centre, grows out of the self and its deintegrates—the archetypes and the ego. This contrasted with the earlier notion that the ego grew out of the impact of instinctual drives with the environment. The two propositions do not contradict each other, however, for each process can go on concurrently with the other.

In this volume I shall concentrate on the archetypes and the self as part of the exploration of the child's 'inner' world; this develops concurrently with the continuous building up of a picture of the outer world, closely tied to reality, and a growing capacity for organized thought, for perception of reality and reality testing.

The maturation processes alter a child greatly as development proceeds, and so confusion can result from thinking of childhood as a single state between birth and adolescence. While it is common usage to talk of a child in this way, it creates difficulties when more detailed studies of growth processes are being pursued. Even a baby, though essentially the same person, goes through many states of mind, very difficult to define in the first months, before he attains unit status at about two years of

---

* The contents of this chapter were first presented in two papers: 'The theory of archetypes as applied to child development, with particular reference to the self', which was read at the Second International Congress for Analytical Psychology and published in *The archetype*. Edited by G. Adler. Basel/New York, Klarger, 1962; and 'The self in childhood', delivered to the Sixth International Congress of Psychotherapy and published in *Psychotherapy and psychosomatic medicine*, Vol. 13. 1964. The two publications have been combined and considerably modified.

3

age. It may also seem arbitrary to say that all these states can be lumped together as infancy, since during the first two years greater changes take place than during any other period of life, yet that is what I and others have found it useful to do. From then on to about seven years of age may be called childhood proper. It ends with the passing of the oedipal conflicts, which then ushers in a period of sexual latency that persists until adolescence. During this period, development may be described as horizontal, for consciousness expands rather than deepens. Adolescence is a separate study and will not be included here. This preliminary statement is necessary to clarify the terms that will subsequently be used.

The Archetypes

The presence and function of archetypes in all age groups of childhood has been a consistent centre of my interest, but I had first of all to overcome a dogma about children current among all analytical psychologists. It is true that in his paper, 'Psychic conflicts in a child', Jung made relevant observations as early as 1910, but he did not then suggest that the archetypal forms were represented in them. Though this study showed quite beautifully the maturation processes in a little girl, yet he was primarily impressed, as indeed were analytical psychologists as a whole, by the effects of parents' unconscious conflicts upon their children. So there could be virtually no significant psychology characteristic of childhood, and the occurrence of archetypal dreams was understood mainly as an intrusion by the parents' unconscious into the child's dream life. A number of observations and reflections led me to modify this one-sided emphasis. They may be summarized as follows:

(a) First of all there was the therapeutic effectiveness of child therapy conducted in child guidance clinics, and observations obtained by studying children evacuated during World War II. The combination showed convincingly that the home, in the past or present, did not alone determine the full range of childhood neuroses, behaviour disorders, psychosomatic diseases and psychoses, not to mention minor disturbances in the development of healthy children. All these could best be understood as due to their being rooted in the complexities of the child's psyche, which contributes significantly to his maturation and to his psychopathology.

(b) Other observations showed me that examples of archetypal imagery could easily be collected by studying children's fantasy, play and dream life, and that its occurrence is related to the child's psychic state. After World War II, I learned that examples of archetypal dreams had been discussed by Jung in his seminars. These confirmed my own systematic collection, which was first published in *The life of childhood* and developed in *Children as individuals* and elsewhere (Fordham, 1957c and 1960). So it can now be taken as established that images representing the self, animus, anima and shadow, etc., can all be observed with ease in children and are not derived only from parental sources.

(c) A theoretical stimulus to my investigations was provided by considering whether any more evidence could be collected from children to confirm or disprove the theory that archetypes are inherited.

Definition of the Term Archetype

In his discussion of Jung's papers collected in *The archetypes of the collective unconscious*, Hobson (1961) listed the various meanings of the term 'archetype' in Jung's writings. His essay has made it necessary for a writer to state how he is using the term.

The general theory was introduced by Jung to account for the regularities observed in the dreams and imagination of adult persons. These were not only experienced as important by individuals but were reflected in the social organizations and in religion and so are an essential element in the psychology of groups. The regularities therefore showed a general and probably a universal distribution, but little had been done by him to show that they could be demonstrated in childhood, let alone infancy.

His massive observations did not take sufficient account of the body-imagery that predominated in infancy, to which I hoped to apply the theory, so it was necessary to re-examine the theory of archetypes conceived as dynamic structures closely related to instinct. I therefore investigated the idea that archetypes might be expressed in impulses originating in

5

neurophysiological structures and biochemical changes (Fordham, 1957), and thus showed that the theory of archetypes could be seen to bring body and psyche together. Jung's thesis as to their bipolarity then became particularly meaningful: the archetypes can be conceived as unconscious entities having two poles, the one expressing itself in instinctual impulses and drives, the other in the form of fantasies. In contrast to the instinctual drives, which are relatively fixed and few in number, the fantasy (or spiritual) component has wide and flexible application.

Transferring this idea to childhood and starting from the spiritual components: the theory of archetypes means that a predisposition exists in the child to develop archaic ideas, feelings and fantasies that are neither implanted nor only introjects. These can be influenced and refined by education which in turn, as in feed-back systems, provides suitable imagery through which the unconscious archetypes can find expression in consciousness. It is on this spiritual pole that parents build when they mediate the culture pattern of the society in which the developing organism is living. So Jung was partly right when he said that the archetypal images showed parental influence; indeed, since parents and educators consciously transmit to their children more or less of the wisdom and experience of the generations of mankind, this must be so. Furthermore, in asserting that the assimilation of transmitted experience involves unconscious as well as conscious dynamic processes, Jung implied that the mechanisms of projection, introjection and identification are here brought into operation and contribute to the growing sophistication of the archetypal images that children manifest. It is indeed the interaction between inner and outer experience that gives to the archetypal images and their associated affect much of their regularity and their typical formal qualities, though they be concerned with extremely diverse experiences. In short, the interaction between inner and outer, between unconscious archetype and environmental components expressed in tradition, causes these to reinforce each other.

None the less, though children become interested in metaphysics and arrive at highly pertinent conclusions, based on their use of logical process and on archetypal imagery and what is transmitted to them, their primary concern is first with bodies,

6

with what they experience of these, and what they can do with them. If, therefore, we are going to trace back into infancy the earliest manifestation of archetypes—and that is necessary in child analysis—it will be desirable to study how the archetype is reflected in early physical object-relationships: we may expect that a body-mythology might best express the infant's experience. Frieda Fordham has done much work on this idea in two papers given in London: one called 'Ruthless greed' (so far unpublished), the other, 'Myths, archetypes and patterns of childhood' (1963); and a great deal of energy has also been directed by psychoanalysts to the study of infancy, partly by using analytic inference, partly by direct observation. Melanie Klein and her followers (Segal, 1964) have developed just the kind of psychology of early childhood that the theory of archetypes would lead us to expect. It is therefore no surprise to find that her close collaborators, Susan Isaacs (1948) and Paula Heimann (1955), both define unconscious fantasy in terms almost identical with a definition of the archetype used by Jung.

Heredity

Can the study of children and infants contribute to the hypothesis that archetypes are inherited? Jung conceived that they were inherited predispositions, so his theory raises the age-old question of how far child development can be considered as a maturational process brought about by the active influence of innate, inherited elements, i.e. the genes, and how far it is the result of nurture.

Through refinement in the definition of heredity, many of the meanings given to the old distinction between nature and nurture have now gone by the board, and it has been realized that no characteristic can be wholly either inherited or acquired. In consequence the science of heredity has become the study of the nature and structure of DNA, and its effect on the development of the human organism.

There is a feature of genetic influence that needs noting here because it has a bearing on the significance of observations we may hope to make about it in childhood. The fact that a characteristic appears early in life does not necessarily indicate genetic influence. If animals are kept isolated until they reach

7

sexual maturity they know, or very rapidly learn, how to behave when released; before this stage in their development has been reached, they do not. Therefore hereditary components of behaviour may be released comparatively late in development, while on the other hand behaviour appearing very early, formerly believed to be inherited, may have been mainly learned.

It follows that the only reason why childhood could be a good period to study the effects of genetic influence is that the structures to be dealt with are simple. Unfortunately by the time one can start analysing children, say by the third year, they are already so complex that analytic inference about heredity has become inadequate and needs supplementing by other means, for instance a combination of observations and experiments. So the question of whether a particular mode of behaviour or experience is inherited or not, while interesting, cannot be easily answered; therefore we are left with the concept of archetypal forms and processes as an operational model. It has so far served us well and shows every possibility of continuing to do so.

Infantile Sexuality

It is my view that infantile sexuality can be considered in the light of archetypal theory for, if archetypes are bipolar, then the theoretical separation between archetypes and infantile sexuality as an expression of instinct could not be justified. It came about because of an irrational value judgement, which asserted that infantile sexuality was of little and the archetypes of great importance.

Hawkey was the first to show the true state of affairs in two pioneering papers written many years ago now (1945 and 1947). In each she demonstrated the importance of the sexual activities of children in relation to archetypal imagery; but one, 'The witch and the bogey', is of quite special interest. She developed there the same theme that Jung had introduced in his revised version of 'Psychic conflicts in a child'. In that paper Jung laid considerable emphasis on the double nature of infantile sexuality, making it clear that he means thereby the germinal roots of its adult equivalent. He says (1910, p. 5): '...while perceiving in infantile sexuality the beginnings of a future sexual function, I also discern there the seeds of higher spiritual functions'. In other words, he recognized by implication infantile sexuality as being, in its very nature, archetypal. This conclusion may be expanded as follows: there is a group of behaviour patterns based on physiological needs and impulses: feeding, in which oral behaviour predominates; elimination, in which the anus, intestines, urethra and bladder expel and control the movements of faeces and urine; genital excitement, which has outlets in masturbation and overt sexual activities between children. The amount of activity and the age at which it is countenanced depend on the culture pattern. When the genitals become special centres of interest, the bodily facts and the custom of preventing children from witnessing birth and sexual intercourse, combined with the inaccessibility of the female genitalia to easy observation, all stimulate speculative, quasi-mythopoeic and logical thinking about these bodily organs and their activities. All this is an important basis for symbolic activity.

The polymorphous nature of infantile sexual fantasy derives mainly from the similarities between different organs and their more or less simultaneous activity. As a result the orifices, mouth, ears, anus and urethra, and the protruding objects, breast, penis, nose, etc., become psychically interchangeable or equivalent. Also, from early in infancy, physiological activities are experienced as predominantly identical with fantasies and thoughts. So arises the 'body mythology' already mentioned, reflecting the relation between parts of or a whole mother and infant.

This formulation involves accepting the psychoanalytic theory of the relation between part and whole objects. According to this, infants first of all experience their mothers and themselves as parts of what will later be felt and perceived as a whole person. Early experience is of a breast, from which they gradually extend their perception to other parts, so that eventually they construct the body-image of a whole mother. A comparable process leads to perception and feeling of themselves as whole beings. In each case the objects, mother or infant, at first either good or bad, come to be felt whole in the sense of being both 'good' and 'bad'.

Only later, as the psyche becomes more organized, do the

archetypes get expressed in the complex spiritual forms that most analysts habitually meet.

Infantile Destructiveness

Unconscious archetypal processes are conceived as both creative and destructive, so examination of infantile destructiveness in this light becomes necessary.

The subject of death was introduced by Jung (1910) at a time when less was known than today. His observations show how the death wishes were then understood. With reference to Anna's statement that if she got a little brother she would 'kill' him, Jung says (p. 10): 'The expression "kill" looks very alarming, but in reality it is quite harmless, for "kill" and "die" in child language only mean to "get rid of", either actively or passively, as has already been pointed out a number of times by Freud.' Here Jung is not referring to the primitive state but to a later and more complex one. It implies that, alongside destructive affects, strengthened by jealousy and envy, there are also strong feelings of love and wishes to preserve the parents and herself. Jung's statement thus involves a combination of love, hate and reflection. Anna had realized that her destructive aims came from only one part of herself and Jung had correctly, though not explicitly, hit on the likelihood of these being linked up with the anal fantasy systems she was revealing, i.e. killing is taken to mean 'getting rid of'.

In these days even destructive fantasies can no longer be considered 'harmless'. On the contrary, we know that they can be very powerful, so that infants and small children can feel intensely afraid of their own death and that of their parents; this is especially so in primal scene fantasies. Their intensity rules out, in my opinion, the idea that only frustration of libidinal gratification causes them. This theory in any case begs the question as to how violent aggression can arise; no, the most severe anxieties arise primarily from the innate violence of affects.

Some psychoanalysts follow Freud in explaining the phenomena by postulating a death instinct. Though the violence of affect is not in question, I cannot accept this theory and think that Gordon (1961) has gone further than others when she understands the fear of death in terms of a threat to the ego. The threat arises from the overwhelming activity of the self, a theme to be developed later in this volume.

The Self

On the basis of his own experience, confirmed by observations of his patients and also by the study of ethnological parallels, Jung concluded that a class of images, expressing totality, symbolizes the self, defined as the total personality, conscious and unconscious. His conclusions involved making a clear distinction between the ego, the archetypes and the self.

Though most of his published data are taken from adults, he also found, in unpublished observations, that the symbolism could be observed in children. It was an observation that I myself had made independently and that has since been amply confirmed. By following and developing Jung's general thesis, I concluded that it was justifiable to assume an original or primal self, a psychosomatic integrate—a blueprint for psychic maturation—from which the behaviour of infants may be derived as they gradually develop and differentiate into children, adolescents and adults.

My reflections on this evidence developed gradually until it became clear that an infant must be thought of as a person separate from his mother, even though a live infant without a mother is not conceivable. At that time this view was revolutionary, though it now seems obvious. It followed that the relation between the ego, the self and the unconscious as a whole could, even in early childhood, be given importance alongside a child's relation to his parents, and thus gave a theoretical foundation for observations on the possibilities for child therapy. It also meant that, very early in his life, an infant had boundaries and individuality other than those constructed during ego-growth. These primitive boundaries come to form the basis for an inner world containing parent figures influenced by the real parents, though mainly imageing the archetypal parents.

It is natural to ask how early these boundaries form. It is not possible to answer that question, but a boundary may very well be thought of as present at conception. There is a common fantasy that, during pregnancy, a mother and her baby live in a special state of intimate fusion disrupted at birth. The true state of affairs is different for, although a mother provides a stable aquatic environment and feeds her baby through the umbilical cord, the growth of a foetus is determined in all other respects by its genetic constitution. Thus there are clearly definable influences at work that are quite different in kind from that of a mother. These may not constitute a boundary in the sense in which I have used the term, but they do provide a basis on which boundaries could form.

The primal self can be conceived as an integrate, a steady state, but if the dynamic systems that we observe later on are to come into existence, it must deintegrate. According to current theory of analytical psychology the self combines opposites within itself; therefore we may assume that when the self deintegrates it will divide into opposites that are psycho-physiological in nature. We may assume, following Jung's theory of psychic energy, that the energy bound in the primary self is neutral and divides into creative and later loving activities on the one hand, destructive and aggressive ones on the other. Each drive follows a partly predetermined pattern and is directed towards objects.

There is another aspect of the dual self's action that needs comment. The drive energies that are released in deintegration produce unstable states. They lead to experiences taking place between mother and infant covered by the term 'primary identity'. It is a matter of observation that these alternate with steady states known as rest, sleep and relaxation. In this early period of an infant's life, the ego being very weak, it is convenient to assume that the self controls the needs of an infant to a large extent, and so those steady states may also be thought of as the manifestation of the self's action: consequently the self may be conceived as a dynamic system that deintegrates and integrates in a rhythmic sequence. It is this that provides for organized differentiation of the self, and underpins the distinction between the external and internal worlds, the self and the not-self.

Differentiation depends upon the acquisition of sense experience. Its beginnings are a matter for considerable controversy, but it must be that images, through which the self differentiates, form largely through the impact of the external world upon the self. At first, there is good reason to believe, the distinction between self and not-self—though real—cannot be perceived and there is much difficulty in describing the condition of a child's consciousness at this time, To help, terms like 'fusion' or projective and introjective identification may be used; they each indicate that a baby cannot distinguish the difference between self and not-self. In subsequent chapters I shall introduce the term 'self-object' to underline the state of affairs.

Self-representations

Data about the self are provided by the study of self-represent-ations. By these I mean any experience felt by the infant and growing child as perceived and felt to be separate from his ordinary field of consciousness, and yet referable directly or indirectly to himself. Much infant experience may be con-sidered as elementary self-representations that develop into the organized and essentially complex experiences known as self-reliance, self-confidence, self-esteem or the sense of being a person with a continuity and identity in space and time. To understand how complex self-feelings emerge or how symbolism refers to the whole self, as expressed in paintings, dreams or fantasy, it is important to consider how a self-representation is related to the whole self.

Early in an infant's life there is probably a wide range of experience that has not reached expression in either image or symbol. It is to include these that the term *representation* is useful. The class of data covered by self-representations—some, of which are vague, others having reached the stage of ex-pression in image or symbol—requires some degree of ego-formation and so some differentiation of the primal self. It is axiomatic that the primal self can never be fully represented in consciousness, though we know that its wholeness can be symbolized. Knowing that a symbol is only the best possible representation of something unknown, from this point of view also it can only be a partial representation of the self. It is a principle that applies to all self-representations; being omni-potent, wishful, or ideal they are obviously partial, though something of the the primary self clings to them. This state of affairs can be formulated theoretically when it is said that they are rooted in deintegrates of the self.

Another feature of a self-representation is that it can be conscious only when there is consciousness of another. And here it is apparent that the body-image, and particularly its surface, is important in the formation of self-representations. In the formation of the image an infant's mother must play a unique part because she is the first 'other' that an infant discovers. Through maternal care she helps her baby to integrate sense data: in innumerable ways she provides the necessary conditions for the baby to do so; the opportunities arise during feeding, sensitive holding and fondling, looking, smiling, singing, bathing, changing nappies and settling to sleep in a cot. Play soon enters into all these activities and this fosters the sense of self. It is through these close physical interchanges that body-image formation is fostered and so awareness of self and not-self, going on to the recognition of the internal and external worlds. Once these are established, a basis is prepared for the construction of symbolic or whole self-representations in their increasing complexity.

Circles and Mandalas

It is easy to observe that children draw or paint geometrical pictures corresponding to those described by Jung as symbols of the self. These are figures, usually circular in shape, having a centre and a varying internal structure (for examples cf. Fordham, 1957c). The way in which changes may take place in children, when painting mandala symbols, corresponds to the more complex results that Jung described; so I see every reason to suppose that the circular patterns can be symbolic images referring to the whole self. For instance, some of these pictures correlate with states of relative stability reached by disturbed children with increased control over the inner world and greater adaptability to the external world. Their appearance is therefore related to ego-development and it is of interest that circular scribbles by infants sometimes correlate with emergence of the word 'I' or 'me'.

It is also possible, through analytic interpretation, to link up these structures with body-image experience. The impenetrability of the circle may correspond to the early experience of parts or of whole body-images (eyes and the main orifices of the body, as well as the mother's breast, are all circular) and there are numerous circular objects, open to the infant's inspection, into which projections can be made. It is not possible, however, to account for the circular imagery by deriving it solely from these perceptual experiences of external objects, because they can become a symbolic image of the self under observable conditions;

To avoid misunderstanding I want to make clear that mandala images drawn by children do not necessarily refer directly to the self as an integrate of all psychic structures. For instance, the magical omnipotence of the circle image is frequently used to indicate a control system, inside which bad and terrifying objects are placed so that they cannot get outside. Alternatively, good and precious objects are placed inside the circle to protect them from often catastrophic dangers outside (cf. Fordham, 1957c).

Individuation

Though a separate chapter will be devoted to the subject of individuation I shall briefly consider it here to put it in its historical perspective. Jung's thesis that individuation occurs especially in later life, after adaptation to biological needs and social requirements has been achieved, suggests that individuation does not occur in childhood. The classical view in analytical psychology is indeed just this, though Jacobi (1967) formulated it rather differently. There she asserted that individuation was a process that required the whole span of a life and that the early processes of adaptation were a necessary preliminary to the later development.

The thesis put forward in this book modifies the classical view but not entirely along the lines suggested by Jacobi. It maintains that the individuating elements in a child, expressed in the progressive integration of self-representations and the way these get built up into the sense of identity and continuity of being, warrant our describing a truly individuating process in childhood, of which adaptation to the environment is a part. To grasp what this means, it helped me to distinguish the experience of the self from individuation. This opened the way to reassessing the material observed in the dreams, play and fantasy of children: symbolic experiences referring to the whole self occur and are assimilated by each age-group through a different experience and understanding of the same self. It is usually held in the classical view that during individuation the ego gives place to the self, which, however, the ego comes to reflect more and more clearly; by contrast, in infancy and childhood the organism aims to establish the ego *vis-à-vis* the world of material reality, the archetypes and so also the self.

With this formulation in mind, a symmetrical theory of the relation between the first and the second half of life can be envisaged: assuming that complete integration, based on realization of the self, is the final aim of individuation, it becomes possible that there is also a state of complete integration in the beginning. It is not realized, nor realizable, at all because there is no ego distinct from the self to perceive it. When the original integrate exists must be left open; it may, however, be conveniently located before birth, which disrupts it—hence the persistent idea of birth as the earliest source of anxiety.

After birth the infant reintegrates before the first feed; anybody who has observed babies soon after birth will see that this idea is plausible. Only after his reintegration does he start, through instinctual activity (deintegration), to make an oral union with his mother in the first feed.

This conception runs counter to the idea that the infant is psychically part of the mother even after birth and so has no identity of his own. It is a thesis usually presented as an unsupported assertion and probably rests on no more than the fact that mothers have a powerful influence on babies; to overestimate it means, however, giving no importance to the infant's own very significant part in the early feeding relationship between his mother and himself.

The next step is to consider in structural and dynamic terms how the child's psyche reaches its differentiated state. My own contribution to that subject began with an earlier volume, *Children as individuals*, and will be continued in later chapters.

Jung's main work centred on the conflicts arising in those who had problems about finding their position in the world and in whom identification with groups, whether political or religious, etc., had proved inadequate. This state of affairs, presented as a feeling that life lacked meaning, led them to find a more individual and radical solution. The schizoid and depressive trends in these patients were clearly defined by Jung and, by concentrating attention on their inner world, he made it possible for them to understand more about the role that self-symbols played in their lives. This concentrated introversion could lead to a solution to their conflicts that he claimed also enhanced their capacity for adaptation.

The cases we need to study to produce comparable data about childhood are schizoid or schizophrenic children, in whom disturbances of the body-images can easily be observed. The manifest difficulty that these children experience in adapting themselves to living in relation to other people, and their difficulty in achieving adequate identification with groups, can also be ameliorated by a comparable introversion, with greater self-understanding. There are quite a number of them who succeed in adapting to their environment and even achieving successes in specialized fields, sometimes even without specialized care. A study of one such case—Alan—will be found in Part Three of this volume.

CHAPTER TWO

Symbolization in infancy

Closely allied to the theory of the archetypes and the self is that of symbols. Because of concentration on their collective, social and historical significance, no attempt of any kind has been made by an analytical psychologist to study how they develop in infancy. Psychoanalysts, on the other hand, having focused their attention on them, have given great importance to them as dynamic influences in maturation; Klein in particular asserted that symbols lie at the root of all talents, while Winnicott gave comparable significance to the transitional object.

It is not my intention, indeed it is not within my competence, to review the complex subject of symbolism as a whole, but only to consider a number of features in maturation that contribute to symbolization in the sense that it is generally understood among analytical psychologists. What then are the essential characteristics of a symbol?

1. In the first place it represents some relatively unknown influence. It differs from a sign in that what is unknown cannot be made fully conscious, nor by lifting repression and uncovering a disguise can the true state of affairs be revealed. Jung's theory of symbols developed naturally in conjunction with his theory of archetypes, for they are represented in consciousness by images that are the only possible medium for their expression. Images are therefore the best possible, in fact the only possible, representation in consciousness of the unconscious archetypal forms.

A characteristic feature of the symbol is the plurality of its possible meanings. It seems to be 'alive' and so acts as a powerful stimulus to consciousness, which strives to exhaust all its contents. When this has been achieved the symbol is said to be 'dead', and the person has assimilated or developed a new attribute for living. Thus, for a small child, parents are known to exist but, their nature being obscure, they are recurrently experienced through archetypal imagery, which is the best

18

possible expression available to the child. But as he grows up he comes to know more about his parents as they are in reality, and he can sort out his fantasy of them from what they are really like. When, at last, he himself becomes a parent the symbolic imagery is no longer required, it has served its purpose, its value is exhausted and it is 'dead'.

2. A powerful source of the plurality of meanings of the symbol is that it combines opposites, transcends them and so unites them and refers to the self (cf. Fordham, 1957). This is its synthetic function, which is particularly required in periods of conflict: indeed it is only when a conflict becomes acute that a symbol becomes truly 'alive'. In infancy there is much conflict but the imagery for it does not, as will be explained, combine opposites until the depressive position has been reached, and so it is not yet symbolic.

3. Thirdly, for a symbolic image to exert its effect, there is need for a sustained attitude that will allow the symbolic value of an image to be recognized: this is called the 'symbolic attitude'. In infancy the degree of sophistication that Jung postulates in this respect is absent: a baby cannot take up a 'symbolic attitude' in the way Jung thought was essential; indeed, if symbolization includes the 'as if' quality, it is not until a child 'pretends' that he can be said to have developed a symbolic attitude. But, none the less, since the deintegrated states of infancy, and the periodically integrated ones in quiet states and sleep, are represented later on in symbols, an infant may very early on develop an incipient capacity to hold its experience in some sense or other.

4. The true symbolic image thus depends for its existence on a certain degree of consciousness and a certain capacity to remember. But since the consciousness of an infant is qualitatively and quantitatively so different from that of a child or adult, it cannot truly symbolize in the first place anyway. Therefore the characteristics of that consciousness need to be considered in more detail.

The theory being advanced here is that an infant's consciousness is at first vague and that objects are only gradually constructed. They are at first self-objects in the sense that the imagery is not differentiated from the objects themselves, and represent the needs of the infant that a mother meets and satisfies; self-objects are organized on the basis of archetypal schemata or models. Concurrently other sense data do not become integrated and are experienced as not-self. They are at first rejected, attacked or done away with in screaming, crying, excreting and other means of evacuation. They form the basis for later bad objects. During this first period of development there can be no symbolization of objects in its developed sense, if only because there is no capacity to sustain conflict between opposites defined as 'good' i.e. self-objects, or 'bad' i.e. not-self-objects, which are got rid of.

It may be postulated that, as the result of archetypal activity combined with manageable instinctual frustration, the first state of consciousness is dream-like, and in it emphasis is laid on the grouping of experiences in terms of their sameness. The self-object tends to select sameness so that apparently very different objects are treated as though they were identical, a characteristic that persists very clearly and will be illustrated at length in the case of Alan (infra, p. 188 ff).

It is this characteristic that gives rise to what Segal (1957) called symbolic equations. She furthered understanding by correlating them with states of ego-fragmentation in which projective identification featured prominently. In a symbolic equation two different images or objects having similar characteristics are treated as the same; only later does one represent the other. Thus, in her view, a thumb or a hallucination is at first experienced as the same as the breast; only eventually do they come to represent it.

Object Constancy

In object-relations theory it is usually assumed that objects are stable in the sense that they are remembered after the person has experienced them. Therefore it is easy to assume that this is the case with infants. There is, however, much evidence that this is not so in the first place, and that an infant has to discover how to sustain an image in his mind so that he can, for instance, remember a feed after he has experienced it. When he develops this capacity he is said to have achieved 'object constancy'; it is an essential prerequisite for symbol formation, which must depend upon the mental capacity to represent experience and sustain the representation of it. I have suggested that, for a symbol to form, experiences must continue and develop so as to achieve a dream-like or hallucinatory quality having archetypal characteristics. Since the archetype, though it creates an image or self-object, does not control its persistence in time, the persistence or constancy of an object, even if it be only dream-like, must be attributed to the development of consciousness.

Loss of the Object

It will by now be apparent that symbolization may be related to the absence of an object and may be important in periods during which a valued object is lost. The affect associated with loss of a loved object is mourning, and much has been learned about its prototype in the depressive position. If successfully completed the result is that the lost object, the breast, comes to be symbolized by a creative, reparative act, restoring the destroyed object internally in imagery and thought; at the same time perception of the real mother is increased. Perhaps the most interesting feature of this formulation is the association of symbolization with destructive fantasies and impulses. In order to create a symbol the self-object must be destroyed, otherwise the urgent need for a creative act is not brought into being: since the breast (as self-object) is destroyed, while the real breast is still in existence, the constructive act can take place only in another way, by abstraction from the object—the abstraction being the symbol.

According to this formulation, the significance of the destructive fantasy depends on the perception that the breast is not only a good self-object, but also a bad not-self-object. The identification of the two in one object changes the nature of the destruction. Attacks only on the bad breast do not bring about a painful feeling of loss, but if, at the same time, the good breast is destroyed then there is experience of loss, which must be made good if the self is to survive.

Transitional Objects

A child who can pretend is evidence for the dissolving of fusion so that self-objects become representational. A special transitional object plays an important role in bringing about this separation.

When an infant has formed his first relation to his mother,

she is likely to have satisfied her baby enough for him to create a breast through deintegration, and to experience omnipotent control over it, though in reality he has none. As a kind of co-operative effort, in which mother takes the larger part, disillusionment then gradually takes place, and a baby starts to recognize his mother as a separate object whom he cannot control. Yet the need for omnipotence persists, so what can the baby do about it? By collecting bits of stuff in his mouth or in thumb-sucking, he discovers a thing that he can truly control, though it is not part of his ego; it is thus the heir to the illusion of mother as part of the self. This then is a very early, if not the very first, true self-representation. It demarcates an area between 'inner psychic reality' and 'the external world as perceived by two persons in common' (Winnicott, 1971a).

Through experience the 'stuff' is put to all sorts of uses and acquires properties it did not have in the first place. It can represent bits of mother, the infant himself, or indeed anything that becomes significant as enlarging his perception of himself in a world of objects.

The transitional object appears at any time between the ages of four months and one year; it lasts a variable time and is relegated 'to limbo' as its contents and meanings become exhausted and assimilated into the area of mental functioning delineated by it: dreaming, play, fantasy, thought and the creative activities characteristic of any particular child. Thus it is like a symbol in having a life of its own, and it can die; it is also truly symbolic in containing opposites.

A feature of Winnicott's account of the transitional object is its importance in discovering the not-ego in a way that is no longer alien, as it was in the first place when it was not-self. It therefore seems that the processes underlying symbolization are important in the construction and discovery of reality, and the distinction between psychic reality and 'external' reality. By deintegration the mother-object is at first made part of the self, an event that provides the stuff of later symbolization. The deintegration endows the object with itself, and because this happens disillusionment can take place, a not-self reality can be discovered and constructed piece by piece. At later stages the perception of the not-self reality includes and needs imagination and symbolization to contain parts of the self previously identified with not-self objects.

Another feature of Winnicott's account is that it seems to describe the root of Jung's discovery of the need for adults to start a process—active imagination—which ensures that psychic reality is defined and perceived as non-ego and objective. The archetypal material that he thus uncovered was related to culture, art, religious experience, and political life, just as Winnicott relates transitional phenomena to play, dreaming, artistic creation and religious feeling.

Symbolic Play

Not all play is symbolic. When, however, Jung settled down to play with stones and pebbles by the Zürich See (1963, p. 168), he intuitively understood that this would open the way to a symbolic life leading to uniting the two parts of his personality in symbols. This he later understood as an essential component in individuation and the discovery of the self.

Jung's searching developed mostly through writing and painting; they are both games in the sense that he relied largely on the spontaneous action of unconscious processes, which he discovered how to set off deliberately; they are play in the sense that their imagery is distinct from both the outer and inner (subjective) worlds. They sometimes contain parts of one or the other but are essentially different from each. Jung expressed the place of his experience by calling the symbolic world he discovered for himself, and which he could show others how to discover, non-ego and objective.

A further common feature between the two activities, play and active imagination, is this: they can be forms of expression that have a validity in their own right and are therapeutic in the sense of making whole. Much of both can express intense conflict or anxiety that arises from the outer or inner worlds but has been split off and repressed or otherwise defended against by the ego. But even these contents can also be near to symbolic matter, or to the place where it is potential.

Material illustrating this thesis, not then made explicit, is contained in my earlier books (Fordham, 1957 and 1969). It first came to my attention when studying children's mandalas and the omnipotent fantasies of a boy. Other examples of it will be found in the play of Alan (cf. infra p. 188 ff) who lived in a 'mad' world—neither his inner world nor the real world but a

23

third one between the two. He exhibited an exaggerated and pathologically disturbed form of normal growth, but through play he grew and found his place in society.

Many years ago I had noticed the similarity between active imagination and play: to distinguish between the two I called symbolic play 'imaginative activity.' It was valuable to approach this subject by making a distinction that emphasized differences in ego-participation. Now, especially since the work of Winnicott, it is more useful to look at similarities, for I maintain that both symbolic play and active imagination stem from the same source: from the self's deintegrative activity.

Symbolic play may be thought of as stemming from the transitional object. It is creative and is the place where progressive individuation and self-discovery are furthered. It contributes to the child's making a living relation with others and expresses the source from which artistic, religious, philosophic and other creative forms of self-expression begin. It is furthermore an activity in which the ego can progressively contribute more and more until, following Jung, an almost complete self-representation can be achieved, together with the extension and enrichment of the ego.

CHAPTER THREE

Religious experiences in childhood*

It may seem surprising, and a diversion from the main content of this book, to consider religious experiences next. Jung, however, identified them so closely with the archetypal forms and with symbolism that I have decided to introduce consideration of them now. I have another reason for so doing: it is often thought that infantile experiences comprise states of mind with which a truly adult person has nothing to do; I contend, on the contrary, that they persist and are progressively integrated into later and more mature living. So in showing that the grandeur, the mystery and the numinosity of religious experience are rooted in infancy and enrich its mature equivalent, I shall make an opportunity to illustrate a thesis about the relation between infancy, childhood and maturity.

Unless the links with the helplessness, the dependence and spontaneity of childhood are maintained, religious experience can lose its true meaning and may become either an empty and formal ritual or merely a rational exercise. 'Unless you be converted and become as little children you shall not enter into the kingdom of heaven' may well have been an intuitive perception of the need for religious life to include the vitality found in children.

Jesus 'called unto him a child' does not refer to a particular or special one. It is significant, therefore, that many children sometimes tell truly impressive numinous dreams and fantasies. I have myself published some in my book *Children as individuals*. They are also to be found in the biographies of religious people. For instance, St. John of the Cross remembered, late in life, a vision of the virgin who rescued his drowning companion, when he himself was a small child. In many ways, however, the most interesting, because it is the most complete, accessible account by a psychologist struggling with religious feelings, comes from

* Previously published in *The well tended tree*. Edited by Hilda Kirsch. New York, Putnam, 1971. Alterations have been made.

Jung himself. In his 'First years', a chapter in *Memories, dreams, reflections*, he shows very beautifully how his intense conflicts over good and evil, expressed in fears of the 'black man' or 'Jesuits', dominated a period in his life. Then there is the impressive dream of the underground phallus which, according to his memory, occurred in his third or fourth year. That is a time when less remarkable children start to have dreams of witches, ghosts, burglars and the like; it is only later that the images become destructive, supernatural or superhuman in size. We need not be too exacting about age groups, but it is possible that Jung's memory placed the dream rather early.

Jung's account of his 'First years' is particularly valuable because it shows very clearly how his active and inventive imagination was shaped and stimulated by the religious idiom of his parents' beliefs and thought. Yet the forms he developed were, in essential aspects, his own; developed out of himself and so giving impetus to the formation of a secret inner life necessary for the preservation of his true self.

Some of his scientific formulations in this context are of extreme interest. He vascillated between thinking of the numinous dreams of childhood as, on the one hand, the child dreaming his parents' dreams that had percolated into him, and, on the other, as pure manifestations of the collective unconscious. These two views are complementary and together give a more likely answer. Thus Jung's dream is just what his mother needed to have dreamt, even though it is also the dream that Jung himself as a child created.

The need for Jung to have a secret may also have stemmed from these dual sources: the necessity to preserve within what was valuable of himself and to protect it from the damaging influence of his parents. Yet secrecy, such an essential feature of his development, is also a need of all children. In general, whether it persists or not depends on quantitative factors; if the parents' beliefs are rigidly held, the secret becomes more important; if they are not, their children may be able to express heretical ideas more openly. A child of about seven years, whom I was treating and will report on (cf. p. 207 *infra*), was one who might, in another age, have become an alchemist. He went through a period of discovering that God was bad. One day in Sunday School, when the teacher was talking about the goodness of God, he protested loudly that it was not true, that God was bad. He was removed from the class, but held to his belief and argued it out with his astonished parents—they had no vested interest in religion, which Jung's parents had, so discussion was possible.

That Jung thought childhood an important element in religion can be gleaned from his personal confession. This can be understood from a passage in 'The child archetype' (1951, par. 275):

> Religious observances, i.e., the retelling and ritual repetition of the mythical event . . . serve the purpose of bringing the image of childhood, and *everything connected with it* [italics mine], again and again before the eyes of the conscious mind so that the link with the original condition may not be broken.

It is not, however, usual to find fully recognizable religious forms in very small children. But these exceptional examples combine significantly with the growing recognition that parent imagos are not only representations of real parents, but are also made up of parts of the self, which creates parents out of itself. It seems likely that the images are indeed mainly self-representations and only later become more and more realistic.

In infancy and early childhood the imagos are representations of body experiences of parts of a person (the phallus in Jung's dream, for instance). But as development proceeds these 'part objects' become built up into a whole body-image. This is dependent upon the child's own increasing perception of and control over his own body mobility. It is also connected with a change in feeling, which starts with there being 'good' or 'bad' experiences according to the pattern of opposites. As ego-development gets under way the baby already develops the capacity to recognize, in his parents and himself, good and bad characteristics. Thus, in the first place, an infant feels there is *either* a good *or* a bad mother—they are not the same person. Later there is a good mother who can *also* be a bad one.

There are other characteristics that are acquired through development from primary integration to deintegration, leading to identity and then later to the reintegration in which the ego participates. On the one hand, there is increasing recognition of external reality and, on the other, of internal processes and their symbolization. Concurrently feelings of guilt and concern begin, and the wish to make reparation for destructive acts and fantasies.

Of course these developments only become stabilized as maturation proceeds. Which ones become firm structures, and how this happens, depends very greatly on the attitude of parents, their surrogates and the culture in which the family lives. Early on, indeed up to the passing of oedipal conflicts, there is considerable plasticity in the functioning of the good and bad parts of the self, and of the mother. At one time one level may be functioning, later on another.

These notes on early stages in maturation mean that nuclear forms of processes and states to be found in religions can be observed without much difficulty: the process of idealization in a relatively timeless state, the vagueness of perception and states of identity, are perhaps the prototype of later feelings of mystery and awe; the pattern of good and evil as opposites or of their interrelation in redemption from sin by the confession of guilt, followed by reparative acts, the true bases for penances, are also easy to observe.

But what of the conception that insists on the importance of the child's freeing himself from his parents? To this theory we attribute many mythological themes centring on the heroic encounter and the battle for deliverance, but what they refer to is not easy to decide. They certainly do not indicate desirable external circumstances, for the sons' and daughters' link with their parents optimally persists throughout the parents' life, and after this is continued in memories; nor can it refer to desirable internal conditions, as the links with the past need to be retained so as to maintain the full integrity of the person; nor to the child's view of the world, which always contains a large quota of what his parents developed and revealed to him. So it can only lead us to understand that its function is to develop a necessary illusion of independence which may (or may not) develop into recognition of individuality. If successful, once this illusion has served its purpose, the child will not divorce himself from the parents but will understand and evaluate them in the light of his own experience, a process that will continue throughout life.

In the main the individuation processes to which I refer proceed without much disturbance. There are, however, definable crisis periods of childhood, up to the passing of oedipal conflicts, which represent a sequence never again experienced in healthy people. There follows the crisis of adolescence, during which acute conflicts again arise, which can sometimes reach the level of a 'normal' psychosis. But it is not till the form of individuation found in later life, when death rather than life looms over the horizon, that once again any serious crisis of value comes about if the person is not ready to make the transition.

Shadow, Anima and Animus

It was in studying individuation in later life that Jung laid emphasis upon the integration of the unconscious as a quasi-religious process. He then defined some of the contents of the unconscious in 'personified' terms—the shadow and the anima or animus. These archetypal figures can all be found in the dreams and fantasies of small children.

At one time I suggested that the order in which they appeared in maturation was the reverse of that in adults, especially those in later life. Since nothing more has developed from this idea, I do not think it can be decided whether it be true or false. In any case it was only a rough approximation, which filled in a gap. It is therefore desirable to start again from some features of Jung's formulations and see whether they can elucidate the subject any further.

In *Aion* he is particularly clear that there are two aspects of the shadow: first, its personal elements that can be assimilated into the ego; second, there is absolute evil, which cannot. It is evident that in maturation the first can be developed only when there is sufficient ego formed and when the child's psyche is structured enough for there to be a repressed unconscious. Without being dogmatic, it would seem that this takes place during and after the oedipal conflicts and their resolution. Absolute evil, however, must refer to a much earlier phase; then infantile affects have indeed characteristics that are most suggestive. They are known to be total in feeling; there is either total and blissful love or else total cataclysmic destruction. It is also in this preoedipal period that projection (and intro-jection) play such a prominent part in the psychic life of an infant and toddler, as I have described it earlier in this book.

At the end of his chapter on the shadow, Jung introduces the

29

subject of 'The syzygy: anima and animus' (1951) by referring to the 'projection-making factor,' which he later identifies with the mother archetype. In reviewing the development of the ego and its weakness in childhood, it is—I think—possible to understand more about the 'projection-making factor'. My assumption of the wholeness of the baby, out of which deintegrates form, having characteristics of the self, leads to the same conclusion as Jung's—that the archetypal forms are partial self-representations (I do not use the term symbol because I conceive a symbol as more complex than an image or representation). In the early relation of the baby with his mother there is probably very little definite perceptual awareness at all, and so what experience he has of the mother—her breast, arms, face, smell, etc.—is conceived to be all one vague perception. The infant gradually perceives and knows his mother through maturation of perceptual processes not yet differentiated from affect. Also in the first place he creates his mother-images out of himself and, in these processes, the discoveries of his mother are more like hallucinations than perceptions as adults know them. Through these the infant reaches his mother and there develops a state of primary identity, sometimes called fusion, so long as his mother is 'a good enough mother.'

At this stage in his development, one might say the baby creates a mother by projection, since the real mother is experienced so much in terms of the infant's self. I would, however, prefer to reserve the term '*projection*' for when the baby's body-image is sufficiently complete for him to experience himself as different from external objects and to feel he has an inner object that can be projected onto the external object.

The earlier state does not have the necessary ego-boundary; the real mother is fused with the part of the baby-self called the mother-archetype. A real mother will seek to meet the needs underlying her baby's view of her and in so doing helps her baby to get into relation with her. If she persists too long in this so that she sustains a state that becomes an illusion about her, then she seems to be the projection-making factor. Jung cites cases in which the real mother does this and continues to reinforce it in later life:

Often a mother appears inside him [her son] who apparently shows not the slightest concern that her little son should become a man, but who, with tireless and self-immolating effort, neglects nothing that might hinder him from growing up and marrying. You behold *the secret conspiracy between mother and son* [italics mine], and how each helps the other to betray life. (1951a).

Here he does, however, recognise the child's part in the conspiracy. But, while cases like this do occur, I doubt their frequency; usually the projection-making factor originates in early infancy, when fusion of the imago with the real mother is the rule. That it tends to be put down to the real mother—where she does not foster fusion—is due to the persistence of this state into the time when boundaries are formed. Projection is a part of maturation that, under good environmental conditions, can be resolved so that, in health, the child begins to distinguish the real mother from the inner mother who has by then become part of his self-feeling.

But what of the animus; why is *he* the 'projection-making factor' in a woman? He—the father—comes on the scene as a libidinal object much later than the mother and after considerable maturation has taken place. It seems to me that the projection can be understood by taking into account the more complex development of a girl. She has two main libidinal objects, while the boy has only one, his mother. For her there is a transfer from the mother to the father, whereas for a boy there is only one object, the mother, to whom his libido is mainly attached. In making her change, the past relation of a little girl to her mother carries over to her father, and so it seems as if he is the origin of projection processes.

Anima, animus and the depressive position

The depressive position is conceived as follows. At first a baby is separate from his mother, then he makes a relation with her based on self-objects. So at this stage a mother is experienced as part of the self. If she impinges on the infant self by not being there or by acting in ways that are foreign to the self, she is treated as alien and not-self; consequently the self-defences are called into operation and she is attacked. The accumulation of pleasurable self-experiences by the baby leads to the construction of good objects while the accumulation of not-self unpleasurable experiences leads to the construction of bad objects that are rendered alien, destroyed or evacuated (the early form of projection).

There is at first no recognition that good and bad objects are related to each other but, as the baby's affective life develops and his ego begins to form, he starts to realize that the good and bad objects can no longer be separated and that the breast-mother is at once good and bad. When, therefore, he struggles with a bad object with the aim of destroying it so as to preserve his identity, he will destroy the good object along with it. When this takes place he pines and very primitive forms of grief and guilt start to form; they lead to reparative wishes and to efforts to reconstruct the breast-mother.

Besides this development the infant ego has grown enough to perceive that the real breast-mother is separate from his mother as archetypal self-image and he is confronted with a person who is not destroyed as her image has been. Therefore the reconstruction, based on the self's integrative action, becomes an internal process and leads to the formation of a symbolic image representing the experience of the breast-mother as part of the self. It is at this stage in development that an inner world begins to form made up of female objects. In the male child they lie at the root of later fully developed anima-images described by Jung and others.

It might now seem that the soul-image of a female must also be female and that she also should develop an anima as well as a man. That this does not happen is due to the way a female child develops. The female symbol becomes integrated in a different way because she can become a mother in the future and so there is a much greater possibility fori dentification with feminine images and her real mother. Whereas a male cannot become a female and so is compelled to symbolize his feminine identifications in inner imagery, a woman treats them as symbols of the self (Jung, 1951). It is when the early pattern of the depressive position is transferred to the father, whom she can never become, that she symbolizes her masculine aspects as the animus.

A feature of the depressive position that will by now have become apparent is that it is the nucleus-experience from which the projection processes can be resolved and through which the anima and animus can become inner functions mediating between the ego and the unconscious.

Ontogeny and Phylogeny

In defining the nature of the projection-making factor, I make the assumption that the past never ceases to influence the present, be it *ontogenetic* or *phylogenetic*. Analytical psychologists have shown mainly the persistence of *phylogenetic* influence, and psychoanalysts have emphasized *ontogeny*. The influence between the two is complicated when considered in detail, but it is not difficult to suggest how they relate positively.

The archetypal forms can be considered as innate structures and processes contributing decisively to maturation; the term 'collective unconscious' is used to mean the archetypes as a whole. There is, however, another sense in which Jung used the term 'collective unconscious'. It was as the complement to the collective consciousness or culture pattern. His thesis may be stated as follows: In any particular culture there are relatively stable systems of beliefs, thought and behaviour, based on religious, legal, ethical conceptions or social custom. These systems never embrace or represent all the archetypal forms; some are left out. Those that remain unintegrated give rise, especially in a highly developed culture, to its shadow, sometimes represented in deviant groups, heresies and mystical development, which complement and may be gradually assimilated into religious orthodoxy. But sometimes they form systems giving rise to several new forms. Jung illustrated this from alchemy as the precursor of chemistry and the psychology of unconscious fantasy and symbols leading to individuation.

If we examine the effect of a culture pattern on infants and children, it is shown to be considerable. Right from the start, in patterns of infant feeding, to the extent that the real mother takes part in child care, in the various techniques of weaning, in the customs that regulate a child's excretory activity and so on, the culture pattern can determine what is done. It is as if it were known that these methods would facilitate the baby's future conformity to what society requires of the individual.

It is transparent that this conformity does not represent all aspects of the self but only a portion of it. Yet my own investigations, and those of others as well, indicate that child maturation starts from a wholeness out of which the ego and archetypal images are derived by deintegration. The unity of the personality nonetheless continues to assert itself and brings about states of wholeness again and again. In particular, the wholeness of the self becomes represented in the ego in the achievement of unit status, which a child reaches at about the age of two.

At the oedipal phase, potentiality for more stable imbalance arises. Then sexual identity is more firmly established than heretofore. Identifications with parents are greatly reinforced and true repression takes place. The basis is here formed for the communication of sexual culture patterns, which play such a decisive role in primitive initiation rites. They are still important today, even though sexual morality is changing and the merging of behaviour by each sex is increasing.

It seems that our present culture includes change more than it did in the past, but this does not avoid one-sidedness. Some of the influences are detrimental, but some alterations are valuable. Intensive study of the mother-infant relation had led to a far more realistic understanding of the essential needs of the mother and her baby. Consequently a large number of mothers benefit as they use the available knowledge. Other results are, however, unsatisfactory, especially when the permissiveness that is rightly applied to the infant-mother relation is extended to all upbringing—to periods when the child's aggression, his primitive and expressive moral feelings need to be brought into relation with a parent who will not allow destructive impulses and who knows how to set firm limits to his child's aggression and destructive activities. Thus a place is made where aggression and violence are safe. With small children permissiveness must be limited, and it is much more important for the future that these limits be well devised and applied. If they are not, then primitive guilt feelings can be overwhelming and result in an anxious, insecure child.

Changes in the culture pattern today have been of considerable concern among analytical psychologists. Before ending I should like to contribute some speculative ideas on this subject.

I have suggested that how children are brought up depends, often decisively, on social trends and custom. Jung has shown us how different cultures emphasize different aspects of the whole person: primitive or archaic man relies far more on projective and magical systems; the east on introverted forms of the self; the west on the development of consciousness, probably derived from the aspiring elements in Christianity.

He also emphasized that it would be a regression to adopt any other than our own cultural tradition.

The progression of society would seem to be in the direction of individuation, which means moral autonomy. As I see it, this would not remove the need for authority nor lead to unlimited freedom. It is rather extra reliance of the individual on discovery, based on recognition of traditional values, which may need modification but not eradication. In a sense there is nothing new about this and indeed it is the characteristic feature of science conceived as a 're-public,' to use a happy term introduced by Polanyi.

I do not think this is the place to enter further into the details of current conflict nor my reasons for thinking, with Jung, that any change in the direction of individuation is to be welcomed. I rather want to point to my contention that individuation processes can be discerned as taking place in the first two years of an infant's life. Therefore how this phase is managed by parents, mostly by the mother, but also by the father through his relation to his wife, is of prime importance in relation to changes taking place in society. If these early stages are successfully managed, then the prospects for the adult are far better than if they are not. In this sense it may be said that the future of our society depends upon the mothers, or rather upon the quality of their instinctive endowment.

It would be unfair and indeed wrong to leave it at that, because the endowment of her child is equally important and, more than this, a mother cannot allow her instinct free play unless her husband also is there participating with her in making a secure and loving home. In addition, the manner in which society enables parents to perform their functions is equally relevant. In the past, as well as the present, it has often interfered. It does not, for instance, allow a husband time off from work in order to be with his wife during, and for a reasonable time after, her giving birth. It is still common for the medical profession to take over the mother during parturition in the often unnecessary interests of hygiene and ensuring safe delivery; and it is still common for custom to replace knowledge.

CHAPTER FOUR

Individuation in childhood*

In *Psychological types* Jung defines individuation as follows:—
'It is the development of the psychological individual as a
differentiated being from the general, collective psychology.
Individuation, therefore, is a *process of differentiation*, having for
its goal the development of the individual personality' and he
adds later on: 'Individuation is practically the same as the
development of consciousness out of the original *state of identity*'
which is '. . . the original non-differentiation between subject
and object . . .'. This state is characteristic of primitive mentality
for it is the 'real foundation of *participation mystique* . . . of the
unconscious state of the civilized adult and of . . . the mental
state of early infancy . . .'. In addition he asserts that 'Identity
with the parents provides the basis for subsequent *identification*
with them; on it also depends the possibility of *projection* and
introjection.' (1921, p. 441). It is the differentiation of the
individual personality out of the state of 'identity' that I select
as being the core of the definition. I shall show how the basis of
it is completed by the age of two. Before doing so, however, I
want to note that when Jung includes 'general, collective
psychology' in his definition he is referring to the social and
religious life of the community constructed by adults. Its
equivalent in infancy is the mother.

Jung thought that the infant psyche is complex at birth and
that the innate archetypal forms are components in its complexity; he recognized individual characteristics from the
beginning of life and understood the powerful effects of the
identity between mother and child; finally he affirmed the
child's capacity to experience the self.

Recent developments have substantiated all these views but
have rendered revision of some of his statements about the ego

* First published in *The reality of the psyche*. Edited by J. B. Wheelwright. New York,
Putnam. 1968. The paper was delivered to the third International Congress for
Analytical Psychology. Minor alterations have been made.

36

inevitable; Jung put ego-formation far too late—between the third and fifth years—and his dating could not have been based upon his own observation; indeed, it seems likely that he took over Freud's ideas, since his dating is very close to one of Freud's; also his theory of the ego's origin, as stated in *Aion,* corresponds equally closely.

The time at which the ego is formed is important for the study of child psychology. The discovery of its early appearance has compelled a substantial revision in much of our thinking and understanding of infants; it has had repercussions on our orientation towards the structure and organization of the infantile psyche; it has compelled a revision of views about the possibilities of infant and child management and therapy. But, in spite of all this, the necessary modifications are congruent with the main body of Jung's thesis, which was so much ahead of its time.

The idea that 'Individuation is practically the same as the development of consciousness out of the original state of identity' is the formulation that knits together what I now want to say. There is evidence to suggest that after birth the infant develops during the first few weeks of life into a state of 'identity' with his environment and particularly with his mother. It is clear that, though the real mother participates, through reactivation of her own infancy used in the service of empathic understanding, this identity is largely created by the infant himself, as observations on the very first feeding patterns suggest. Thus identity is not the primary state of an infant, but develops because of fusion by the infant with his mother. It can be inferred that the infant can only fuse with those parts of his environment that correspond very closely, and at first exactly, to his own needs; indeed any event that does not correspond with his immediate needs may not exist for him. I take this as confirmation of the theory that the primary unity of the self exerts a powerful conservative influence. Such a state of affairs, although persisting into adult life, also rapidly modifies itself, probably in the first few weeks of life. It is superseded by the phase in which object relations are essentially omnipotent, as archetypal forms deintegrate more clearly out of the self and gain expression in perceptual imagery.

At this stage of archetypal object relations experienced as omnipotent, there is no knowledge corresponding to a person having an inside or an outside. Experience is first of all in terms of the fusion of part-objects: mouth and nipple are one total experience. Soon total experiences are separated into those that satisfy and are blissful, and those that are frustrating and rejected—the first equivalents of later good and bad objects have been experienced.

In the early months of an infant's life it is essential for him to obtain sufficient good and satisfying experiences so that there may be a foundation for later separation. If this happens, development does not occur so much through pain as through the primitive equivalents of sadness and grief, balanced by knowledge, pleasure, and satisfaction in new achievements. But there is another necessity for separation to become a rewarding development: the infant must feel himself to have a boundary between himself as an object and others as objects. This happens for certain at about six months, though it may happen earlier, between the fourth and fifth months. It is the first step in individuation.

In all the early period before the ego-boundary has formed, the infant's mother gets drawn into the state of identity required by the infant. During the first few months and also for some time afterwards, the infant is viable so long as suitable conditions are provided. The mother-infant unit must be the most important object of study and here Jung's intuition about children as a whole, now known to apply most of all to infancy, i.e. before the second year, is on the mark. But, all the same, nobody truly separates from his or her mother; indeed continuation of union makes possible recurring and fruitful fusion with others in later life. The states of identity can be grown through, can recede into the background, but they never disappear. In them are the roots of the anima, the superordinate personality, and the persona.

Turning to studies made of the mother and baby unit, observations over several years on the couple in longitudinal studies have shown how, besides fusion, infants display their own individuality from the beginning, while showing clearly that their behaviour is an expression of the mother's unconscious fantasy as well. The course of development is therefore largely defined by the child's individual capacities in relation to his mother's emotional and fantasy life.

Observational studies must be of particular interest in that they give immediate data relevant to the idea of the infant being part of the mother's psyche. They show that this is only true in part; each infant expresses his individuality within the fantasy and behavioural systems of his mother, but from the start he also develops behavioural, perceptual and fantasy systems characteristic of infancy and peculiar to himself. They evolve, deintegrating out of his primary unity or self, and through new integrative acts they form the basis of the child's ego, his experience of his self-system, and his continuity of being in space and time.

This thesis can be studied through the observations of mother and infant, of the way the infant reacts to his mother, of infants who are disturbed by their mothers, and of infants who are *reacted to*, who are met and related to by their mothers. Then it can be observed what happens when the infant becomes dependent on his father and later gains independence from him also as he develops his capacity to do things for himself. Before the second year the infant has accomplished sufficient mastery over his mouth, hands and arms to feed himself, over his legs and body musculature to walk and run about, over his eyes to look, and over his anal and urethral spincters through which he gains control over his faeces and urine; he has developed a sense of his surface as distinct from his mother's body; he has discovered his skin, and he has discovered that there is an inside and outside to himself, and that he can exert control over what goes in and what comes out.

The days have passed when an infant was thought about as either a physiological unit or an auto-erotic being; instead, he can be seen as a psychosomatic unity relating increasingly to the object with his libidinal and aggressive drives and his developing imagery, using his thoughts and feelings to deduce and evaluate his experiences. All the developments sketched here in bodily terms are filled in with a wealth of psychic activity; indeed, the bodily achievements are the correlates and sometimes the expression of psychic operations. The achievement of a state of physical control over bodily activities means that the two-year-old has also grown psychically out of the state of identity into a separate being with an individual unit status.

To consider further some of his mental and emotional achievements: he has emerged from a primitive, ruthless way of living to become a person who can show concern for others;

he has known love, hate, fear, grief, sadness; he has the basic rudiments of a conscience, and he has developed a clear distinction between internal and external objects, which he evaluates as good and bad; he distinguishes an inner world from the outer; most interesting of all, he has developed true symbols that express his inner life.

By the age of two, therefore, an infant can achieve every essential element in individuation in the sense Jung could have accepted. I say this advisedly, although he studied a different age-group and therefore represented it very differently.

The process described does not require anything more than ordinary good mothering, but it may be remarked that many sophisticated methods of infant care seem almost designed to do all they can to retard the process. Of course unit status is extremely vulnerable and can be thrown out of gear or seek inappropriate and pathological expression if mishandled, mismanaged or misunderstood. Yet even then it can reinstate itself if given a chance and hence its growth and elaboration can be resumed, whether the failure occurred in childhood, adolescence, adulthood, or in the second half of life and during old age.

CHAPTER FIVE

Primary self, primary narcissism and related concepts*

In this and the next chapter, I shall bring the concepts that have been outlined into relation with comparable formulations by psychoanalysts. In the process essentially Jungian ideas will be thrown into relief and amplified.

In *Children as individuals*, I developed a concept of the primary self; in this paper I shall relate it to Freud's theory of primary narcissism (Freud, 1914, 1916–17, 1920, 1923, 1924, 1940). But before doing so I shall discuss another and seemingly opposed speculation, which states that a baby is psychically part of his mother; it represents the only other significant though radically different view of the earliest psychic states in infancy.

Observations on Babies

Before we go into each theory further, here are some simple facts about a baby that are easily lost sight of though essential to keep in mind. After birth he spends the main part of his life sleeping or dozing, but from time to time he wakes up and requires attention. The infant may awake hungry and cry, or his mother may anticipate his need and pick him up before he signals to her. When she does so and holds him, he will reach an upright position; then he initiates approach behaviour, a sequence of movements that lead, with his mother's help, to taking the nipple and sucking it.

Next ensue a number of physiological activities that convey milk to his internal organs. After a time that may vary he is satisfied, the physiological processes underlying hunger are no longer active and he soon goes to sleep again.

---

* Previously published in *Journal of Analytical Psychology*. **16**, 2. 1971. Modifications and additions have been made.

Another situation that starts after birth is bathing. It includes muscular activity with legs and arms, being washed and having his skin dried. Soon bowel movements begin and the baby's interaction with his mother is extended to all the interchanges that centre round diapering. From now on an increasingly complex active and reactive situation is set up, having a wider field of application. In this development play features prominently, his activities are none the less periodic and the baby sleeps most of the time, say 18 out of the 24 hours in a day, without dreaming; there are no reliable data suggesting that he dreams, till about eight months.

It follows that the baby is separate from his mother's body for most of the time and that when he is with her he is actively reacting to her. It may be said that she is represented all the time in the conditions she provides—cot, clothes, blankets, etc. —but these are stable instruments of care that provide an environment approximating to the intra-uterine state. They are not part of the reactions that centre on breast-feeding, bathing and diapering.

INFANT AS PSYCHICALLY PART OF HIS MOTHER

In this nuclear sketch I have made observations about processes known to be complex. The feeding situation itself is complex and in infancy sleep covers a number of different states, the study of which has already proved interesting. They are described in various ways but, although some degree of agreement has been reached about the data, no satisfactory conclusion about the physiological or psychological processes underlying them is as yet possible (Robinson, 1969).

I shall, therefore, leave these interesting topics on one side and now take up in more detail the postulate that a baby is psychically part of his mother in the first place. It asserts that though a baby is physically separated from his mother at birth he is psychically part of her (Jung, 1928—par. 106). It follows that he only achieves separation gradually, after an unspecified number of years. I would stress that this theory has not been developed in detail nor expressed before as concisely as has been done here. I believe, however, that my formulation states its sense.

The view, as known to me from analytical psychologists, is derived from the following observational sources:

(a) The passivity of infants.

(b) Experiences in analysis reconstructed as fusion between mother and infant (Newton, 1965).

(c) The fact that the analysis of mothers often benefits their children (cf. Jung, 1926; Wickes, 1966).

(d) The experimental work of Fürst (1909)—a pupil of Jung's—on identifications between members of families and Jung's (1909) development of her thesis.

(e) The fact that some children's dreams can be referred to their parents' affective but unconscious life (Jung, 1926; Wickes, 1966). In addition it was discovered that children, in relating themselves to the unconscious affects of their parents, are compelled to act them out in their own lives.

None of these observations refers directly to the earliest state of an infant in relation to his mother; but they may reflect aspects of it and so they will be considered in some detail.

(a) To assert that a baby is essentially passive is to underestimate his equally important activity. The fact that most of the time he is sleeping or dozing, either in his cot or in his mother's arms, does not mean that he has to be stimulated or seduced out of this state—as Freud postulated at one time; it is a view that wrongly suggests that only the mother creates the activities centring on feeding; though of course it is true that her sensitive reactions are all-important.

It seems also true that her influence is mainly through her unconscious and that she certainly contributes to the formation of the infant's first feelings about himself in many subtle and far-reaching ways. It would be a mistake, however, through overemphasis of her importance at every stage in infant maturation, to overlook that right from the start observations show how active the baby is in creating for himself a relation to his mother (Call, 1964). Indeed it is possible to look at the feeding mother as a passive instrument fitting in with her baby's approach and attachment behaviours so as to satisfy his needs.

(b) Next, to consider observations on fusion: analysis of them shows that they are of two kinds.

1. States in which there seems to be fusion because the baby has not discovered how to distinguish between himself and the parts of his mother with which he comes into contact.

This state of affairs is not, however, the baby being part of the mother's psyche; it is rather a perceptual state of the infant. It says in itself nothing about the mother herself except that she has been there providing conditions for the 'confused' perception between subject and object to occur.

2. States in which the mother's affect gets mixed up with the infant's. Mother and baby both have the same affect, such as a feeling of blissful union or violent and disruptive confusion, at the same time. Yet fusion involves the mother becoming part of her baby's affect as well as the other way round.

It is justifiable to hold that these states occur very early on, but simple observation of infants shows that they could not take place at the start; they must therefore be developed. Indeed, Mahler, who pioneered in this field (cf. Mahler *et al.*, 1955), claims that the symbiotic phase, in which fusion is included, is not established till the third month.

(c) As regards the observation that analyses of mothers benefit children, it must be noted that the examples given in the literature are of quite mature children; as far as can be ascertained they are in the oedipal phase or later, i.e., four years or more. Given, however, that this is quite often true, it is also well established that psychotherapy can be usefully conducted with children themselves from about the second or third year onwards without alteration in their mothers' psyche (cf. Klein, 1932). If a small child is only fused with, or not differentiated from his mother, this would not be possible. Furthermore, psychotherapy with children under six years of age is known to be particularly productive because of the maturation potential they exhibit.

As far as the literature goes, it is probable that the improvement that children often show when a mother becomes a better mother (as the result of analysis) is due to improved techniques of infant care or to the modification of identifications developed in the course of maturation. Identifications are not, however, there at the start, but are the result of maturation. Yet it was the effect of these that impressed Jung in his early years when revealed in association experiments and case histories of adults. To conclude these thoughts, it must be stated that it is not always true that a child improves when his mother becomes a better one, for he may reveal how disturbed he is and so appear worse.

(d) The subject of identification is more complex now than it was thought to be when Fürst and Jung developed their ideas, especially because of this difficulty of sorting out identification from introjection (if this be possible at all). In crude terms, however, and that is all that is necessary here, it is established that identifications influence a child's attitudes; longitudinal studies show this very beautifully (cf. Colman, Kris *et al.*, 1953). But clear identifications do not show up till months of development have taken place and they do not refer to the earliest states of infancy. Therefore it is confusing to apply the theory of identification, as used by Jung, to the first weeks or months of life.

(e) The last category considers dreams and a child relating to the unconscious of his parent. These are part and parcel of the complex relations between a child and his parents and, in the literature, refer to developed states. If they are to be referred to early infancy they need refining. The importance, however, for child development of his relation to his parents' unconscious cannot be in doubt; the way in which a mother's responses to her baby, or her lack of them (covering death wishes (Bettelheim, 1967)), or her forcing herself (as breast) into the infant, can foster or disorganize his need-motivated approaches, is especially worthy of note.

The Infant as Unconscious

The idea that the infant is psychically part of his mother is implicitly combined with another one: the infant is said to be unconscious. In current usage the term *unconscious* is ambiguous: it refers on the one hand to a negative state in which perceptual functions are not giving rise to conscious awareness and on the other to a more or less organized and partly inherited system of structures referred to as unconscious archetypes.

It would, I think, be very daring to assume that an infant is *not* capable of any conscious experience and there is some indirect evidence in favour of there being ego-consciousness in very early situations. Right from the start, i.e., after birth, and indeed while still in utero, the infant (or foetus) reacts to

45

stimuli. That the responses involve reflexes and neural discharges of an organized kind is certain and it would be much more logical, since reflexes involve afferent stimuli, to assume that at least some of them are accompanied by perceptual experience, however vague.

It is worth remembering here that the foetus is recurrently subjected to stimuli and especially noises. One source is from the mother herself: the movement of food substances along the intestines, leading to defaecation, and the heart beat. It is known that noises from outside the mother's abdominal wall reach the foetal auditory systems and result in motor activity.

Recently there have been serious attempts to investigate this difficult topic and, while there is not yet a psychology of intra-uterine life, there is now a growing consensus that there are organized perceptual ego-functions at birth. Some think they must be inchoate, as Spitz's ingenious reconstruction, combined with infant observation, suggests. He postulated a 'cavity experience' which, he writes, is 'the perceptual combination of the tactile sensation of the nipple in the mouth, plus the cutaneous sensation of being cradled at the breast, and the simultaneous visual perception of the face' (Spitz, 1960, p. 86). Others conceive—following Freud—that perception is hallucinatory and again there are some, like Call (1964) who, basing their deduction on infant observation in the first days after birth, believe that quite complicated secondary processes involving memory and choice are brought into operation in the first few feeds.

The other use of the word *unconscious* brings for consideration the inherited endowment of an infant and the degree to which it is organized. There is still little agreement on this matter, though the evidence of ethologists (Bowlby, 1969; Tinbergen, 1951) supports the idea that there are organized mechanisms giving rise to behaviour patterns discharged upon the receipt of suitable sign stimuli. The theory of archetypes, which presupposes organization, is in line with this view (Fordham, 1957a).

There does not now appear to be any basis for assuming that infant endowment is unorganized, but this view is still current, so needs mentioning. In it—according to Freud (1914)—the ego, cathected by undifferentiated libido, becomes a 'reservoir of libido' and then sends cathexes out into the external world.

Thus is formed the idea of an original libidinal cathexis of the ego (narcissism); some of this cathexis is later given off to objects, in much the same way as the amoeba extends or withdraws its pseudopodia into or away from its environment. On this view the libido is not object-related but is a libidinousness attached to objects and given out by the ego.

As to the nature of early object-relations, Anna Freud (1960, p. 56) writes. 'There is no libidinal exchange with the object as there will be in the later stages of true object–love (loving and being loved). Instead, one-sided use is made of the mother for purpose of satisfaction. The object . . . is drawn wholly into the internal narcissistic milieu and treated as part of it to the extent that self and object merge into one.' This formulation does not deny, indeed it suggests, organization in the first place.

I have introduced this discussion because it amplifies the part played by the infant's mother in establishing the mother-infant couple. The views held on this topic vary with the views held about infant endowment. If this be conceived as primarily unorganized then the way is open to think of him as psychically part of his mother, who creates the feeding situation and gives form to the infant's patterned life—sleeping, feeding, excreting, bathing, etc. Like most views in this difficult field, there is something to be said in its favour, but its extension is no longer tenable, though at the same time it is self-evident that a mother contributes to the patterning of the infant's actions and reactions. On the other hand, if the infant is essentially an organized being with specific needs of his own, then what she does is also, and perhaps mainly, a meeting rather than a creating of them.

To end this section of my chapter: the conception of the infant as psychically part of his mother focuses on a number of states worthy of serious investigation, but it must be borne in mind that if this concept were really true all the work on infant study would be pointless and indeed fallacious.

The theory that an infant is psychically only part of its mother in the first place implies that he has no individuality of his own and has so little to support it that it is relevant to enquire why it attained the status it did. The enquiry cannot be developed far in this context, but it is worth noting that it may derive from a mother's *feeling* that her child is part of her. In handling the mother–child relationship the feeling is usually expressed in terms of maternal guilty omnipotence. It expresses the conviction that everything that goes wrong in her child's development is her fault. This is really a subject on its own and so may be left aside for more detailed consideration elsewhere; a large literature has, however, grown up round this subject and reference may be made to Pollock's study (1964) on the symbiotic element in mother–infant interaction: symbiosis, he contends, may be global or focal; it may be appropriate and part of healthy development, or inappropriate and lead to psychoses or neuroses. Symbiosis, however, covers much more than states of fusion; it covers all the times that a mother and baby are mutually dependent on each other.

In contrast, indeed in seeming opposition to the idea that the infant is basically part of his mother, stand the theories of primary narcissism and primary self. I will consider each under a separate heading, starting with primary narcissism.

PRIMARY NARCISSISM

To explain the reason for the libido's turning away from reality, Freud (1914) was led to postulate that the libidinal state of the infant was primarily narcissistic: without his mother seducing him, the external world would have no attraction and the infant would never establish any attachment to his mother at all. Like the view that an infant is part of the mother from the start, this is a speculative reconstruction and was recognized as such by Freud. There is only one piece of direct evidence that can be used in its support: the predominating tendency of the infant to sleep.

Evidence for Theory

The theory that sleep is a narcissistic state derives from application of libido theory which states that since there are no evident object-relations, the libido must be applied internally. Freud (1900) contended, however, that the egotism found in dreams was a derivation of primary narcissism, though when he wrote 'On narcissism' he did not believe there was any ego at birth. Later, in 1937, he conceded that there could be; this view has been widely accepted by psychoanalysts and, as a result, the theory has become tidier and topographically easier to picture, i.e. the infant's early object-relations are derived from primary investments of the ego by libido.

After introducing the death instinct Freud (1920) revised his position. Adhering to his dual-instinct theory, which accords with the conflict situations found in the analysis of children and adults, he worked on a theory of fusion and defusion of libidinal and aggressive energies. Thus the primary state was thought of as a fusion of them and so was masochistic (Freud, 1924). It is interesting to note here, in parenthesis, that this theory *corresponds* to, but is not identical with, my own idea of integration and its correlate deintegration.

The other empirical sources for the theory of primary narcissism were the omnipotence of thought among children, their narcissistic object-choices—reflected in later sexual perversions—and their egotism. There were in addition the narcissistic neuroses, especially schizophrenia, and also the behaviour of patients suffering from organic disease and hypochondria. Theoretical objections to the speculation have been worked over by others, especially Balint (1968), and I will not repeat them because to analyse the conditions from which the theory is derived is far more important. When we do so the result is not favourable. There seems little doubt that the narcissism of patients with organic disease and hypochondria, like the narcissistic object–choice in sexual perversions, is secondary.

This leaves us with the theories of schizophrenia and of the omnipotence of thought. Freud held that schizophrenic patients differed from the neurotic ones in one essential aspect: they could not develop a transference because the whole of the libido was applied *not* to object cathexis but to the ego, producing omnipotence of thought.

Since Freud formulated his ideas it has been shown that his observations, if they are not definitely false, are subject to doubt. In particular the transference in schizophrenia is not now held to be absent, but (on the contrary) to be particularly intense and delusional (Jung, 1946; Rosenfeld, 1965; Sechehaye, 1951; Searles, 1965, etc.). It had been difficult to elicit with the techniques of psychoanalysis Freud was using, because—I suppose—the necessary associations were too dangerous to reveal. So the theory of primary narcissism does not receive the support it did at one time from observations on schizophrenia and the other 'narcissistic neuroses'.

The omnipotence of thought found in small children remains for consideration. Anna Freud (ibid.) writes that it is due to 'cathexis of the self' without saying whether it is derived from primary or secondary narcissism. She probably does this because of serious doubts among psychoanalysts.

Related to the omnipotence of thought are the egotism and auto-erotism of the child. These characteristics have been over-emphasized, and indeed, with reference to the former, Bowlby (1969, p. 354) states on the basis of his own studies on infant observation and an extensive review of the behavioural literature, that 'There is, in fact, no reason to think that a child is any more egotistical than an adult'. There is reason to suppose he is more auto-erotic than the adult, but not so very much. Though Freud (1914, p. 77) thought auto-erotism was the first state of a baby and prior to narcissism, yet even an infant is not wholly auto-erotic, any more than he is wholly narcissistic. In these respects adults and children are quantitatively rather than qualitatively different.

The more and more the concept of primary narcissism is reviewed in the light of increasing knowledge of babies, the less and less credible does it become—yet there is something about an infant's naive feelings to which this term narcissism is particularly appropriate. He seems self-contained, self-centred or somehow whole and, one might say, in love with himself. So it would be unfortunate if, in rejecting the grounds on which the intellectual conception is based, the feeling content of Freud's hypothesis were lost.

The impression of wholeness, which I have nonetheless preferred to develop, was expressed to me very well by a mother. She said she felt her baby's future was contained in him and she only had to make its emergence possible. The tendency to cast aside such impressions as invalid on intellectual grounds must be resisted. They are not stated very precisely, but they are common and I believe it is wrong to ignore them, even though they are not adequately expressed in terms of behaviour and have not sufficient objectivity to satisfy those who hold that objectivity alone is 'scientific'.

Ego Ideal

Freud postulated that the ego ideal derived from primary narcissism as follows: 'The subject's narcissism makes its appearance displaced on to this new ideal ego, which, like the infantile ego, finds itself possessed of every perfection that is of value . . . what he projects before him as his ideal is the substitute for the lost narcissism of his childhood in which he was his own ideal' (Freud, 1914, p. 94), and this takes place 'with the intention of re-establishing the self-satisfaction which was attached to primary infantile narcissism but which since then has suffered so many disturbances and modifications' (Freud, 1917, p. 429).

The important point in Freud's construction is to introduce a particular instance of a general proposition: earlier states of mind influence and motivate the formation of later structures. From this position the particular instance Freud took amplifies a thesis that has been current among analytical psychologists without, however, receiving the attention it deserves: the self, it maintains, is the dynamic principle behind the development of ego-consciousness.

Just how this took place had not been considered until the theory that the self deintegrates to form ego-nuclei had been introduced. The nuclei integrate partly through the development of thought and partly through the integrative action of the self. In as much as the primary state of the self becomes idealized it would be represented as the ego ideal as Freud expresses it.

Alternatives to the Theory of Primary Narcissism

The theory of primary narcissism has been subjected to criticism by a number of psychoanalysts, two of whom have put forward alternative views that can now be considered.

Balint (1968), who has analysed the metapsychological and empirical data in detail, points to contradictions in Freud's metapsychological constructs. He concedes that they have been commented upon and in part resolved by Hoffer and Strachey (*cit.* Balint), but he is not satisfied and then considers the clinical data. He correctly grasps the nature of Freud's theorizing as attempts to express or explain clinical data in abstract meta-psychological terms. This makes it clear that metapsychological ideas need not be consistent since the changes reflect different assessments of the ever growing observational data.

After critizing the data much as I have done, Balint rejects primary narcissism by showing that the data on which it is based are wrong. He then goes on to assert that it is false to say that in infancy the external world is not cathected: it is only necessary to change it, i.e., remove the foetus from the uterus, to realize that the environment is essential. This is evidence, he says, for very intense cathexis of the external world by the foetus and infant after birth.

In the place of primary narcissism he substitutes primary love. Object-cathexis, he maintains, is very intense but there are no definable objects, only a vague or nebulous experience of them which slowly comes to clear definition. This theory has the advantage that it accounts for the infant's active approach behaviour to his mother and the active part he plays in breast-feeding. It does not, however, seem plausible to suppose that there is anything like the global object-cathexis before birth that Balint proposes. After birth there is good evidence for object-cathexis during waking periods, but only reactions to noise, thumb-sucking, swallowing amniotic fluid, etc., suggest anything like cathexis of the environment during embryonic existence. Balint's special use of the term 'cathexis' is not satisfactory and the biopsychological argument that he uses to support it reminds me of the daring, often intriguing speculations in which biologists have always loved to indulge. I think here of Gaskell's *Origin of the vertebrates*, various theories of vitalism and more recently de Chardin's (1959) brilliant quasi-mystical philosophizing.

Nevertheless the idea of the infant's first cathexis being active 'loving' and seeking satisfactions, rather than his having to be seduced out of his primary narcissism, is in line with conclusions arrived at from infant observation and experimental data on early modes of perception. In addition Balint's insistence that all narcissism is secondary is in line with clinical observations.

The second critic I want to consider is Edith Jacobson (1964). She also rejects primary narcissism; she considers it particularly in relation to the oscillation between love and hate that implies the existence of a pool of neutral energy. Freud held that the pool was built up in the ego by a process of neutralization, but Jacobson rejects this and instead postulates a pool of primarily neutral energy within a primary self out of which differentiated libidinal and aggressive drives emerge. This state of affairs, following Freud, would mean a fusion between the death instinct and eros and the ego, which then corresponds to the concept of the wholeness of the self in analytical psychology in that there is a union of the ego with opposites—a state that in later life becomes symbolized.

I should like to add here—to avoid confusion—that, in psychoanalysis as a whole, the self is conceived as that part of the ego that refers to self-feeling. They have followed Hartmann (1950) who distinguished between the external object and the self. This is not in line with my thinking, for it appears to me that it is better to contrast the external with the internal objects. Only a few psychoanalysts postulate a primary self in the sense of Edith Jacobson. For her, self-representations—omnipotent, wishful and realistic—are partial representations of the self and in this she comes close to my position, though hers does not allow for symbolic whole self-representations.

PRIMARY SELF

The data on which I began, in 1947, to elaborate the hypothesis that the self is a primary datum were as follows (cf. Fordham, 1957b):

1. The occurrence of self-symbols in the fantasies and dreams of children.
2. A few observations on the use infants made of circles in relation to the formulation of the word 'I' or 'me'.
3. The observations collected together under the heading of infantile omnipotence.
4. The way mothers treat their babies as persons.

Subsequent support came later from:

1. Discussions with others studying children who favoured the idea of the wholeness of babies.
2. The work of Rhoda Kellogg (1969) on children's finger paintings and drawings, especially the fact that mandala figures lead to the formulation of a body-image in pictures.
3. The realization that the thesis would under-pin data about child analysis.

4. The recognition that it provided a theoretical foundation for the therapeutic value of regression.

My hypothesis assumed that the self is not reducible to anything else and that the symbols depicting union of the opposites in children and adults represent, in complex and elaborated form, a state from which the infant began. I first suggested the term 'original self' for the first self-integrate in infancy so as to contrast this state of affairs with the later symbolic self-realizations (symbols) to which Jung and others have directed so much attention.

In parenthesis I would like to remark that on my thesis current conceptions of the mother as a 'carrier of the self' are wrong. Besides pandering to maternal narcissism, they deny the basic separateness of the infant from his mother. But if this view were stated to mean that to the baby his mother is a part (deintegrate) of the self, then I would demur because in essential respects the infant creates his mother in the light of his own needs and she therefore represents a part of the infant self.

It is not observational data only that make the concept of the original self seem valuable. Without it a basis is lacking for the persistent recurrence of integrative states that form the root pattern for the infant's growing independence of the mother. So much of his life is dependent upon her devotion and care that a powerful motive for independence is needed; an important one can be found in his original psychosomatic unity in which he is not related to his mother. Growing independence can therefore draw on the earliest state of separation which, in spite of states of fusion and identity, persists throughout all maturation.

The primary state of unity gives rise to, or forms the foundation of, later self-representations (cf. Fordham, 1969) in the ego, expressed in the achievement of unit status (at about two years) and a sense of self, carrying with it vague feelings of continuity of being and identity. Earlier derivatives of the self are those in which the infant treats his mother not as a separate object but as part of himself—one form of fusion experience. This, it may be held, is due in the first place to the global nature of perception; but in itself it points to the organization of perceptual input into a unitary perceptual system which only later deintegrates into specific and clear perception.

Into this gradual process may be fitted the early hallucination-like experiences in which subject and object are not differentiated, the later omnipotence of thought and the formation of the ideal self-representations of various kinds, benevolent and malevolent, comprising ultimately the population of fairy tales and myths.

CONCLUSION

In comparing my own thesis with Freud's, I am struck by the similarities. Freud postulated primary narcissism, which I express as the primary wholeness of the infant. That he called it narcissism was in line with the sexual theory of libido. At first he did not allow for the probable existence of any ego at all, but later on did so. When, later still, he introduced the death instinct, along with its sexual opposite, the primary state could no longer be called narcissistic but masochistic and comprised a fusion of opposites and the ego. This might be a definition of the self, to replace the term masochism with something more appropriate.

But it is not only this theoretical convergence between my theory and Freud's—becoming closer and closer as psychoanalysts develop it—that struck me. One feat that Freud achieved was to understand how *the primary state becomes the motive force* for constructing the ego ideal and infantile omnipotence in which, according to my conception, the self is represented so that each may now be termed ideal and omnipotent self-representations.

The use of the term deintegration—corresponding to instinct defusion—is valuable because it keeps in mind the essentially interrelated activity of functional systems of adaptation and provides a basis for ego-formation and for the periodic integration of ego-fragments into what we know later as an organized ego-structure.

But there remains the difference in the theory from the self as formulated later in psychoanalysis. To analytical psychologists the self is a concept that expresses the wholeness of the human being, and the division of the whole into body and psyche, as we know it in adult life, is a development of it. The self is therefore more than a psychological concept and as such it cannot be directly observed. It can, however, be inferred, represented symbolically, and is a relevant postulate in infancy in the ways I have outlined. In psychoanalysis as a whole, the self is that part of the ego that refers to self-feeling and only Jacobson postulates a primary psychosomatic self, as far as my investigations go. Self-representations—omnipotent, wishful and realistic—are conceived by her as partial representations of the self, with which I agree, with the proviso that some of them refer symbolically to the total self as Jung maintained.

CHAPTER SIX

Maturation in the first two years: Freudian and Jungian concepts compared

In this chapter I shall relate my position to developments in psychoanalysis since Freud. My reason for so doing is that much work has been done by psychoanalysts on the first two years of life, and much of what I have discovered has been stimulated by their researches.

But there are difficulties upon which I feel it necessary to comment before doing so. I have no direct personal experience of what either a classical or a Kleinian psychoanalysis is like, so when reconstructing a patient's history, I do not know whether the way I treat my patients is much or little like the way psychoanalysts treat theirs. This introduces one source of error that is inherent in discussions between analysts but, if it is sometimes hard for Jungian analysts to understand each other, it is far more difficult when they refer to members of other schools. So when I refer to particular features such as the depressive position, or individuation, there are practical implications that cannot be worked out in detail and can only be theoretically related to. Let me take an example: Klein based her ideas on the death instinct and this theory informs her work, giving conviction to her interpretations. When, therefore, I say I accept the depressive position but am very uncertain about the death instinct and think of it in relation to defences of the self, this will mean that I cannot give an interpretation with the same conviction as Klein and, further, that my views will influence the details of my interpretations and so the material produced by patients.

In spite of this, however, there are data that Kleinians have recorded and that I have myself observed. I often confirm the relation between persecutory and depressive anxiety, and note that, if the former is converted into the latter, then the stage is set for a radical therapeutic alteration. In this respect I can agree that Kleinians have correctly formulated clinical data, but when I go on to consider depressive-position theory I incorporate it into my own frame of reference. Whether the change that takes place is beneficial and advances knowledge is a matter that concerns me but of which I am not always sure. As, however, it is my aim to develop Jungian ideas to see where they lead, I am not primarily concerned with whether they do or do not agree in detail with those of Klein, but rather have the hope that they will. All the same, if I conceive that ideas and observations of psychoanalysts have advanced knowledge by the use of analytic methods, I accept them. The attractiveness of Kleinian formulations to any Jungian struck me soon after I started to investigate and treat children. Her ideas evidently presupposed that an infant was a complex organism and, further, the theory of unconscious fantasy systems, present from the start, was close to the idea of innate archetypal forms. Therefore I approached Klein's writings predisposed to accept much of what she said.

Today I regard many of the *patterns* defined by her as valid, especially the splitting processes (based on deintegration) with concurrent idealization and persecutory anxiety going on to feelings of pining, at the destruction of the good object, leading to reparation. I also think that these two stages are related to the move from symbolic equation to true symbol-formation, the development of the rudiments of an inner world and concurrent growth of reality sense. I consider that this sequence depicts an early individuation process and progresses from states of identity through projection to self-realization. I also recognize the usefulness of the concepts of projective and introjective identification. I doubt, however, the dating of these processes and think it mistaken to understand all of them as due to ego-functioning. It is not easy, with a Jungian background, to think about these patterns as brought about by processes in the ego. The difficulty is one that has exercised others, and especially psychoanalysts, some of whom have engaged in lengthy critical assessments of Klein's ideas, observations and reconstructions. The question that may be asked is: why is so much attributed to the ego? This can be approached by considering the views of other psychoanalysts. When Edith Jacobson conceives of energy in the primal self as undifferentiated, she indicates that primarily the self is virtually unstructured. This idea derives from classical concepts of the id, which consists of instinctual undifferentiated libido; so any structure that can be observed will be attributed to the ego, but how early is this in existence? Klein, following Freud, assumed the existence of the ego at birth.

Within psychoanalysis, criticism of Klein depends on the state of the ego in infancy. It is held that the processes that she believed to take place in the baby are not possible because the infant ego is much more rudimentary than she conceived it to be. Consequently her reconstructions are projections of more sophisticated fantasies back into childhood. One such Kleinian construction is the early onset of the primal scene, corresponding to the conjunction in Jung's conceptions, and so the father is brought into object relations much earlier than had usually been assumed. This thesis has been widely criticized. If, however, it be assumed that a baby's object relations are built up out of his experience, plus a capacity to draw inferences, the early onset of primal-scene fantasies cannot be rejected out of hand. Even without applying archetype theory it is quite possible to construct a plausible hypothesis about how the father comes into the picture, starting from what a baby can experience. In the following construction I shall put adult knowledge in brackets. A baby knows about bodies or about what adults would see as parts of them. He knows fairly soon that a thing can go into a hole and that this produces sensations that give pleasure and satisfaction (adults know that the hole is his mouth and the thing is his mother's nipple). He also knows that there are other less reliable sensations connected with things coming out of him: these produce relief but can also be frightening and uncomfortable (these events are known by adults as evacuation of urine and faeces.) At first these experiences are not much located in space, nor can the baby know much more than the sensations in themselves (this is the basis for what is known as confusion of zones, but it is important not to assume that an infant finds it confusing), but it will not be too long before he gets the impression of an interrelation between things going in and out of each other, and gradually this becomes differentiated into what is self and not-self (mother and himself). Later on he gets to know that there is another kind of thing that picks him up and does not produce sensations of substance (milk) going into him (this is father, with no breast). He also observes that these two things (mother and father) are sometimes together in a way that is like the being together with mother, and he will notice that they are sometimes together in a way that excludes him. Is it too much to believe that he concludes that they do together what he and his mother do together? If he does, then there is a basis established for a primal-scene fantasy. I do not want to say that this construction is true but it is possible, and so the early onset of the primal scene is possible. It will not be a knowledge of what adults know as intercourse but it will grow into that in the course of years.

The subject is complex, but the processes Klein defined, or which have been elaborated by her followers, may be correctly described but wrongly understood; in short, she is trying to express in terms of the ego processes that are the result of deintegrations of the self, not essentially attributable to the ego but to the way in which the opposites in the archetypal unconscious interact.

Winnicott, who accepted Klein's work with modifications that need not be entered into here, introduced ideas having a distinctly Jungian flavour, true and false self being perhaps the most striking. Besides this he introduced the mother into the Kleinian system in a way that was decidedly reminiscent of Jung's formulations developed by Frances G. Wickes. All that he said was, however, more precise than anything from either of these authors, and so he advanced knowledge of the infant-mother relationship in a way that is acceptable.

Now to consider the psychoanalysts who have studied ego psychology: by 1937 Freud had postulated that the ego was inherited and so present at birth, and this was taken up and elaborated by Hartmann in a number of abstract meta-psychological papers. These I have not fully understood and I find them almost impossible to read, so I will merely observe that they exist. Under Hartmann's inspiration, but also as a result of Anna Freud's work, the theory of the ego has developed considerably.

A number of other interesting hypotheses have since been developed that are relevant to the Jungian position. Mahler, in particular, develops the idea that an infant's life at first 'centres on continuous attempts to achieve homeostasis' and consequently a baby attempts to discharge tensions by urinating, coughing, defaecating, sneezing, spitting, regurgitating, and vomiting, etc. The baby cannot record anything but visceral release of tensions, there are no representational objects and no boundaries to the self. This conception derives from Freud and illustrates the consequences of thinking of a baby as initially an unorganized id on which mental attributes are constructed through impact with the environment. For Mahler object relations develop comparatively late and have nothing of the precision that Klein and others—including myself—believe is possible. For instance, she says that it is only between the second and fourth months that a baby develops a 'dim awareness of the need-satisfying object' and can behave as though he and his mother were a single omnipotent system. At this stage the baby has created an essentially hallucinatory and 'delusional' system in which the baby experiences himself and his mother as a unit with a common boundary.

The next phase in development is, according to Mahler, to be called the separation-individuation phase, during which the infant detaches himself from his 'delusion' and concurrently from his real mother as well, to become a toddler. Graphically Mahler says: 'This separation-individuation phase is a kind of second birth experience . . . a hatching from the mother–child common membrane. . . . This hatching is just as inevitable as is biological birth.' (Mahler and Goslinger, 1955, p. 196). In this Mahler's view coincides essentially with my own, in spite of the difference about earlier development; I cannot, however, agree to the idea of a common boundary between mother and infant which, though graphic, does not seem to have clinical application and so is redundant. In other respects her construction of the infant's relation to his mother is useful because it makes clear that very early on the infant establishes a system of object relations with his mother in terms that can be related to clinical experience. Ideas of this kind are needed because of the tendency to think of fusion as a state in which mother and infant are at one with each other.

As part and parcel of her individuation hypothesis Mahler develops the concept that 'The aim and successful outcome of this individuation process is a stable image of the self . . .' (ibid, p. 197). She makes it clear that she thinks a stable image of the self is established by the toddler stage and that it 'depends upon successful identifications on the one hand and on the distinction between object and self-representations on the other.' (ibid, p. 197). Thus, by about two years of age, an infant has developed a feeling of what he is like and has an identity of his own. I would add to this that this has always been there from the start and that the infant has by this time become aware of it. How much is this self-concept, that has been considerably developed in psychoanalysis, like Jung's and the applications of it that I have developed?

It was first introduced into psychoanalysis by Hartmann, who distinguished between external object-representations and the self. Since then a large literature has grown up and is in the process of developing. Edith Jacobson expounded it at length. She starts from the idea of a primary self, with a pool of neutral energy from which libidinal and aggressive drives derive. It does not seem quite clear why she selected the term *self* for subsequently she conceives it, at least in its representations, as a part of the ego, which allies itself with other mental structures, the id or the superego; thus arise qualities of the self-representations—wishful, idealistic or realistic. Thus the term *self* is restricted to the persons's experience of himself as what he is, what he wishes to be, or what he ought to be; it is not used to refer to anything that cannot be truly known in Jung's sense, but that can be and is represented in symbols found among the dreams and fantasies of small children.

Some of the elaborations of the self as part of the ego have, however, been useful: for instance, the relation of self-feeling to the development of the body-image from representations of part objects. With this concept in mind, the idea of ego-nuclei of the kind that I have postulated, following Jung—as Edward Glover did too—fits in well. In psychoanalysis the separate ego-nuclei are brought together by the cathexis of perceptuo-motor systems and identification, so there is no place for the essential contribution of the self as conceived in analytical psychology. Having said this, I should add that psychoanalysts do recognize the concept of the whole person and know that the person does recognize himself as a person who, in the midst of change, is yet always the same self. This implies a central core that is stable. Jungians could reconsider the symbolism of the self in the light of these formulations, but such an approach has so far been resisted.

From this brief survey of the subject, it is clear that there is a great deal to be worked over in considering how the theoretical position of analytical psychologists relates to developments in psychoanalysis. I have made an attempt to do this in my book *Children as individuals*.

Methodology

The first steps in gaining deeper insight into the first two years of the infant's life were dependent upon reconstruction. Freud, deeply impressed by the narcissism of the child, evolved a theory of primary auto-erotism leading to narcissism. Jung, more impressed by the lack of ego, started from the vaguer idea of the infant being unconscious and in the power of his mother. Neither of these views was based on more than very cursory study of children. In a metaphorical style they express something of the nature of infants and their relation to mothers though they both lack sufficient precision and clinical evidence.

Since Freud and Jung first formulated their ideas, a very considerable amount of knowledge has been assimilated, based on the following approaches:

1. The application of analytic ideas to the interpretation of the behaviour of small children and infants.
2. Observational studies on infant behaviour and longitudinal studies in which babies and mothers have been followed up into childhood.
3. Studies of infants that have added experiment to simple observation. These investigations have not found global concepts of much use and have sometimes developed special languages of their own, as Piaget, for instance, found it necessary to do.

If there is any result from these researches, it is to show that a baby is a complex person and that the old generalizations are becoming more and more precarious. Thus it is no longer useful to draw the conclusions that the baby is unconscious or that he is capable only of narcissistic love.

The ideas I have expressed in this chapter are related to global concepts about infancy, and to beliefs about what sort of person a baby is. I have shown how, by assuming the inheritance of archetypal processes, it becomes easier for Jungians to understand some of Klein's theories, which can be better explained by introducing our concepts and particularly that of the self. In addition, I would apply the term *individuation* to processes already going on in childhood, in much the same sense in which Mahler uses it.

Because of my views I am predisposed to accept some researches and not others—for instance, I find it very hard to believe that conditioning or learning theory is of much importance, though I know that by using sophisticated experimental techniques rather interesting conclusions are being arrived at. But as behaviour-theory is undergoing considerable modification, it may be hoped that their findings will provide information against which analytic theory can be checked.

APPENDIX
to Chapter 6

Two reviews of books by psychoanalysts

The self and the object world. By Edith Jacobson.

My first impression of this book was exciting. Jacobson's subject features prominently in analytical psychology, for Jung had studied and defined a symbolism of the self in increasing detail over the last forty or so years. An additional predisposition to be interested derived from my application of Jung's thesis to childhood and to the origins and development of the ego; here was evidence that psychoanalysts were taking up the subject, bringing their greater resources in manpower and disciplined analytical method to unravel a difficult field of study that I had found extremely rewarding.

The volume, however, soon caused me considerable difficulty for two reasons: firstly, though many of the concepts were understandable, others needed translating to fit the frame of reference with which I was more familiar; secondly, there was a complete absence of the kind of empirical symbolic data that Jung had taken to represent the self.

This made me decide to start this review as if Jung's observations had not taken place, and to proceed as if I knew enough of psychoanalysis to make myself comprehensible. As occasion arises I can then introduce ideas current in analytical psychology. In this project I have been much helped by Jacobson's lucidity, which makes me confident that if I blunder it will not be her fault.

I shall start by recording *first impressions* and shall say how this book stimulated me on a first reading.

1. It is a good book, well set-out, persuasively written, and well arranged.

2. The book contains the kind of psychoanalytic metapsychology that I have thought becomes too often so remote from

everyday analytical work as to make it a special discipline of its own. Reading on made me revise my attitude and led me to study quite a lot of her references, particularly those in *The psychoanalytic study of the child*. Some of what I read was valuable and I began to reflect actively about the place and use of theory (metapsychology?).

3. The book showed in a very clear way, which I had not met elsewhere, how the relation between pre-oedipal, oedipal, and post-oedipal developments of the child are conceived. This helped me to understand: (*a*) Freud's theories of primary narcissism and primary masochism. Both ideas had been impossible for me to assimilate before, and I can now see why: I had arrived at an idea of the primal self, and this blocked my understanding. Jacobson spelled out my quandary, and I can now grasp what is meant and where to place the two concepts. And (*b*) why there has been so much conflict over the data and theories described and elaborated by Melanie Klein. It still seems to me fussy to bother so much about whether the 'precursors' of the superego are to be called superego or not, and I very much missed any discussion of the transition that Klein discovered between the early splitting processes and the depressive position. This is surely relevant to the emergence of symbol formation and object constancy. There were clear statements of the importance of accumulating enough good internal objects for a firm sense of self-esteem to develop, but the account of how this comes about is thin.

4. The book contains an illuminating discussion of the ideas about the self and identity in psychoanalysis. I was interested to find reference to Erikson's thesis, because it comes near to Jung. I learned that from a sociological and historical angle, realization of the self could be '. . . caused by the breakdown of the value systems of the past . . .' (p. 25), an idea long current in analytical psychology.

5. The author's use of the term 'self-representations' left me puzzled; several times I could not understand to what they referred, nor what was their relation to the primal self.

6. The book contains many points with which I found myself in close agreement. Let me set down some of them and my rather immmediate comments:

(a) There is the idea of a primal psychosomatic unity from which psychic structures develop. The importance of this idea, which can only be supported by inference, since the physical pole of this unity is not and cannot be represented, is two-fold: first, it defines the self as more than a psychological entity; second, it gives a theoretical basis for possible later whole self-representations. I could not find the second idea developed in Jacobson's volume.

(b) Out of the primal self, whose energy is neutral, two drives—libidinal and aggressive—are differentiated. The drive theory involves an abstraction from empirical observation—a point that I felt was not clearly enough made—and I did not feel certain whether Jacobson intended to dissociate these drives from vestigial structures or not. Empirically, drives are built in right from the start with patterns of behaviour in which an object is implicated.

(c) The need to differentiate between the self and its representations is evident if confusion is to be avoided. A comparable distinction is found in analytical psychology between the archetype and its image. Unlike its psychic representation (image) the archetypal substratum to the self is only accessible indirectly to perception by the ego.

(d) The acceptance of individuation as a part of child development. This conclusion I had been reaching with trepidation. I am quite sure from the way it is discussed that Jacobson had not any idea of the difficulties I had encountered. She simply did not know that *in analytical psychology* individuation was supposed only to occur when 'the usefulness of identification ends' (p. 28).

So much for first impressions. There are rather close agreements that encourage me to embark on a more critical discussion.

I am not convinced that Jacobson has succeeded in making her terminology consistent, though she assures us that she has made every effort to do so (p. 62). She says, and I agreed after much trouble, that her usage is mostly understandable, but some goodwill and mental ingenuity are required rather too often. As the difficulties cannot be due to negligence, therefore, they may be due to the theory's not being sufficiently worked out to accommodate the data to which she is referring.

It is possible, though I could not decide, that her tendency to confusion arises because she operates with hypostatized concepts: the self, the superego, the ego, etc. This might have been why she sometimes equates the concept self with the actual self-representation. While I agree with using hypostatized concepts as abbreviations, there are well-known pitfalls in doing so and I am not convinced that Jacobson exercises sufficient care in an area where it is of particular importance.

Returning to the main issue: Jacobson's distinctions between wishful and realistic, bodily and mental self-representations are certainly clarifying, but she does not seem to understand that a self-representation is a perception by the ego of those *parts* of the total self that are accessible to internal observation. This comes out clearly if we consider those self-perceptions that come into prominence in states of stress and crisis and in relation to demands being made on the child. It makes a great deal of difference how a child estimates his capabilities in relation to frustrations imposed by parents. He must rely on a partial self-representation that will give the relevant internal data to the central ego. ('Central ego' is here used to meet the idea of the self-representation being *part* of the ego systems (p. 29).) This representation is very incomplete and varies according to the child's situation. During development an agglomeration (pooling) of such data results in a sufficiently reliable self-representation being laid down for the person to develop a sense of identity, self-reliance, self-confidence, and continuity of personality. This increasingly complex organization must include bits of id or superego being organized into a special part of the ego.

It is evident that most self-representations are hardly related to the primal self at all. Put in this way, i.e. that Jacobson's self-representations are partial and contain only a bit of the total self, we can understand many of the contradictions in her expositions, e.g. 'physiological discharge . . . on the self' (p. 9), or the self being dominated and controlled by the superego (p. 54), etc., both of which are out of the question if the self is the total psychosomatic unity.

A similar quandary is met in analytical psychology, and it led Jung to formulate different and incompatible definitions of the self: the totality definition in which the self comprises the 'ego and the unconscious', and another later one in which the self is defined as the central archetype of order, i.e. an unconscious datum. It is of interest that the later definition correlates rather closely with Jacobson's reference to 'the centralized, regulating power of the superego' which 'may be properly called an indicator and regulator of the entire ego state' (p. 133). It is of further interest that Jacobson thinks that the functions of the superego are increasingly taken over by the ego, just as Jung contends that the ego increasingly mirrors and approximates to the self.

But, even though Jung himself thought that the superego was the closest of Freud's concepts to the self, this does not mean that they can be identified. It would go beyond the scope of this review to discuss this rather fascinating subject, but I can perhaps make a brief comment on it by introducing some more critical ideas on Jacobson's thesis, which will reveal something of the theoretical ideas that Jung's work has made possible for me.

Jacobson does not spell out sufficiently the theoretical consequences of postulating a total psycho-physiological self from which psychic structures, each becoming gradually autonomous, emerge. Clifford Scott started to develop them when he defined his idea of the body scheme. He clearly understood that the self was a transcendent postulate of which the mental apparatus was a part only.

Except where she refers to psychosomatic disorders, Jacobson studies psychic aspects (self-representations) *in*, not *of*, the total self; she does not press home the inevitable conclusion that each psychic structure, whether it be the ego, id, superego, or reality principle, is part of the total self. If the self is the total organism (including the body), clearly it will be necessary to include the ego and the reality principle as parts of it, even though the reality principle is designed to record the activity of external not internal objects. Jacobson seems to have been led astray here by Hartmann's distinction between the external object-representation and the self. The better distinction is between the external object-representation and the internal object-representation. This point seems to be on the point of clarification through Sandler's work on object-representations.

The perception of objects as internal or external is a complex and very considerable achievement. It did not exist at the start in infancy, and was not to be discerned in the primal psychosomatic self. Indeed, only when psychic representations are established can we begin to consider the question of whether

69

they refer to internal and external objects. Further, what is internal and what is external is at first vague and is used confusingly in the literature, as Jacobson has observed. Much unnecessary vagueness can be dissipated, however, if we ask a rather specific question on each occasion: to what is any particular datum internal or external? It is only too easy to assume that the primal self pattern is translated directly to the growing organism, which consequently develops into having an inside and outside like a bag, with objects inside and outside it having no insides and outsides of their own. This is fallacious, for each object will have been experienced as having an inside and an outside. First, there are part objects; later, whole objects; the breast, out of which comes milk, can be emptied and objects like faeces can in feeling be put into it. Only when the whole body-image is complete is the ground laid for considering what is inside it and what outside the ego-system as a unit. Only when the whole body-image is experienced can we get clearly whole-self-representations expressed in symbolic imagery, based on the existence of a surface structure with the objects external or internal to it. I did not succeed in discovering any reference to such imagery. Without it we can only observe a group of self-representations, changing during development, referring more and more to the sense of individual identity, in which the person is felt to be continually separate and distinct from others. These may be conceived to draw on one or all of the psychic structures; each is a part of the self and varies according to which separate structure is most relevant or which combination is most appropriate to the situation in which the growing child finds himself.

To make my meaning clearer, suppose we construct a working classification of self-representations in a fairly well-developed person. They would be divided as follows:

(i) Data that are not felt to refer to the subjective self at all but to external objects

(ii) Those *felt* to refer to 'the self', i.e. that refer to the inner world of internal objects. Many of these feelings are derived from the ego, others from the id, others from the supergo and again others combine elements of each

(iii) Those that refer to the total integrate derived from the primal self, but are represented to the ego indirectly or felt as a kind of nucleus standing firm and giving rise to the feeling of being 'the same in the midst of change'. If Jung is right this feeling can be represented symbolically and the symbol refers to the total self.

I should now like to consider Jacobson's discussion of Erikson's idea that 'identity formation begins where the usefulness of identification ends'. This was certainly the content of Jung's idea, and is remarkably close to his concept of individuation. Jung observed individuation in older people (though he seems also to have concluded, without publishing this conclusion, that children individuate also) where identification with social groups or culture patterns no longer gives sufficient meaning to their existence. The answer was found by the adults re-evaluating their lives by each one's finding the meaning of it within himself. This might be expressed by saying that each one needed to relate his previous partial self-estimations to a more and more total self-representation.

Jacobson goes rather farther into adulthood than is usual in psychoanalysis, and so somewhere towards meeting Jung. Her researches can be taken to suggest that the individuation process that Jung described is continuous throughout the life of an individual. Her formulation clarified for me an idea that, though identifications are essential, should they exclude individuation the result can only be an automaton made up of numerous identifications without individuality. According to the age of the person the form of individuation must be different, and the methods used to foster it correspondingly variable. In some people it is certain that individuation can best be initiated by techniques that lay bare the infantile roots of their disorder and so go on to make possible a more true or more realistic assessment of their whole self. This is only hinted at by Jung, though he contended that individuation is an on-going process in adults and a continuing process thoughout life.

The high expectation with which I started out to read this very condensed and stimulating book ended with a sense of disappointment. I had learnt a lot about a part of the ego called 'self' by psychoanalysts, little about the self as understood in analytical psychology. It may be that such an attempt to make occasional links between the two is all that can be done now but it would be sad if that turned out to be all that was possible.

The self and autism

There are trends in analytical psychology that want to construct a special relation between the ego and the self. They can be formulated in this way: the ego reflects the self. If this be so, Jacobson must be on the way to illuminating the nature of the self as well as the ego and we may therefore expect further developments from clarifications of this fascinating topic.

On human symbiosis and the vicissitudes of individuation. Vol. 1. Infantile psychosis. By Margaret S. Mahler.

Margaret Mahler conceives that individuation takes place in childhood. She has defined a number of interlacing but none the less distinct stages in maturation culminating in the separation-individuation phase.

Her primary assumption is this: an infant's life at first 'centres round continuous attempts to achieve homeostasis'; consequently a baby attempts to discharge tensions by 'urinating, defaecating, coughing, sneezing, spitting, regurgitating, vomiting . . .'; and because of his inability to record anything but visceral release of tension and because there are no representational objects and no boundaries to the self, he cannot distinguish his own activities from the 'mother's ministrations in reducing the pangs of need—hunger'. This phase is called normal autism.

From the second month onwards, and culminating at around four to five months, the baby develops some 'dim awareness of the need-satisfying object' and so he behaves and functions as though he and his mother were an omnipotent system—'a dual unity within one common boundary'. This is the symbiotic phase which is a creation of the baby and is a 'hallucinatory somatopsychic omnipotent fusion with the representation of the mother and in particular the delusion of a common boundary of the two actually and physically separate individuals'.

The separation-individuation phase culminates at the toddler stage at about two-and-a-half years. It takes place when the infant detaches himself from his mother and is a landmark in the development of identity-experience based on the self. 'The infant's inner sensations form the *core* of the self. They seem to remain the central, the crystallization point of the "feeling" of

self" round which the sense of identity will become established
. . . The sensori-perceptive organ—the "peripheral mind of
the ego", as Freud called it—contributes mainly to the self's
demarcation from the object world. The two kinds of intrapsychic structures form the framework for self-orientation.'

These conclusions are based on studies of child psychoses, of
infant observation and longitudinal studies of healthy infants
and mothers in 'well baby clinics, etc'. Mahler's working out of
phases in development has therefore gone beyond uninformed
speculation and even if they be later modified, as no doubt they
will be, they yet have a degree of reliability that can be made
use of. It is interesting to note that her observations show
changes at three to four weeks, two months, four to five months,
seven months and ten to sixteen months, etc. These orientating
dates help in mapping out the extraordinarily rapid changes that
take place during maturation.

Mahler's work started from observations on a group of
psychotic children; she pioneered in this field, bringing into it a
degree of order that others had failed to achieve. She distinguished autistic from symbiotic psychoses though she had
modified her initial view that each could be clearly differentiated. She now holds that the two psychoses may interlace
but with one form predominant.

The two psychotic constructions employ definable defence
processes—deanimation, dedifferentiation, devitalization and
drive fusion and defusion; in the aggregate they are called
'maintenance mechanisms' conceived as 'restitutive attempts of
a rudimentary or fragmentary ego which serve the process of
survival'.

There are in these findings many points of agreement with
my own constructions; but I regret her use of the term 'symbiosis', which is liable to produce unnecessary confusion. It
gives the impression that she is discussing the mutual advantages
that the two parties gain from each other in their interaction.
Mahler adequately explains that she is not using it in this sense
but as a metaphor; yet all the same the term will give a wrong
impression to anybody familiar with biological usage which
can be and has been usefully employed by Pollock in the
description of mother–infant interaction.

Then there is her assumption that the infant 'attempts to
achieve homeostasis'; this leaves out his part in actively

establishing breast-feeding. As she 'finds it most useful' to adhere to Freud's speculations about primary narcissism her idea is presumably a biological version of that psychological concept. She believes that it is physiology and not psychology that will contribute most to our understanding of early infant behaviour; but if it is to be physiology, to introduce a word like 'attempts' (which is surely a psychological idea) seems inappropriate. In addition, physiologically an infant surely functions not only in terms of homeostatic equilibria but also through disturbances of these followed by their re-establishment. She also accepts, in the very early period of infancy, the idea of a stimulus barrier introduced by Spitz; this seems to derive from the 'bird's egg' metaphor of autism introduced by Freud, which lacks evidence and seems unnecessary; it leads to therapeutic practices to be considered later.

With these reservations, there are many useful and revealing formulations in the first chapter. The second is on 'infantile psychoses', in which she introduces the part mothers play in the symbiotic phase and there is a later chapter on 'Prototypes of mother–child interaction'. There are numerous clinical examples. Some of the accounts are extremely moving, especially the case of Violet, a musically gifted autistic child.

Mahler's ingenious therapeutic practices are based on her conception of two kinds of psychoses and are the logical outcome of her thesis. Treatment in groups, in special nursery schools or centres of education, is undesirable at first; intensive and long personal treatment is needed before any attempt is made to introduce a child into a group.

In the autistic psychosis the child must be lured out of his state (autistic shell) with the help of inanimate objects because he is intolerant of direct human contact, especially physical touching, cuddling, etc. The objective is to lead him on into the symbiotic phase.

Once this has been reached the objective changes: the therapist must fit the child's hallucinatory and delusional system in any manner prescribed by the child. In this stage verbal interchange, music, feeding, bodily contact feature among the wide variety of approaches that may be indicated. An especially interesting technique developed out of the observation that there comes a stage when the child goes to seek his mother while in a nursery school or when a treatment session is in progress; so Mahler decided to include the mother in the therapeutic situation when the child gave indications of needing it: she found that the mother could help the therapist by informing him about features of the child's behaviour and particularly his sign-language, which is often very difficult to decode. In return the therapist could help mother to understand the nature of her child's needs and instruct her in how to manage the symbiotic phase.

The third stage in treatment consists of reliving traumatic experiences, which can only take place when individuation is far advanced. There are no follow-up studies, but these will be included in the second forthcoming volume. I would have liked, however, some longer case studies so that the changes that took place could be seen in more detail.

Today what Mahler says is not new because so many of her findings have been integrated into common knowledge and have been confirmed and developed by others. My own much more (numerically) limited studies lead to conclusions that often correspond rather closely with hers; in particular I have worked for years in the belief that child psychoses are best treated in the first place at home, even though there is a risk that the whole process will be interrupted by the child's parents; *Dialogue with Sammy* is an excellent example of how this takes place—Sammy's mother replaced her son in therapy.

Then came Bettelheim with his striking results from the institutional treatment of autistic children. His cases, however, received an unusual amount of skilled personal care, but even under these circumstances parents would interrupt treatment by removing them from his institution. I regret that Mahler uses educative procedures so much and lays such emphasis on luring the primary autistic children out of their supposed shell. It blurs her thesis, and the alternative that they might come out of it, given good conditions and analysis of the psychotic super-structure, is not considered. It has yet, however, to be demonstrated convincingly, though Bettelheim suggests it.

The field of child psychosis is still wide open to further study: Mahler has worked out a model and so has furthered capacity to define the area and to conduct treatment with more precision—there are clear examples of how her frame of reference makes otherwise daring manoeuvres quite simple and straightforward.

The self and autism

This is a rich, thought-provoking, scholarly book. Its good bibliography gives access to the growing literature on individuation in small children in a way that will, I hope, engage the interest of all analytical psychologists.

Note:

The review of *The self and the object world*, by Edith Jacobson, was originally published in the International Journal of Psychoanalysis, **46,** 4, 1965; that of *On human symbiosis and the vicissitudes of individuation, Vol. I, Infantile psychosis*, by Margaret S. Mahler, in the Journal of Analytical Psychology, **17,** 2, 1972.

CHAPTER SEVEN

Infantile autism: a disorder of the self*

An outline theory of the self and its relation to individuation has been developed and the ground has now been laid for considering theoretically a particular disorder of childhood.

Pioneering work has been done in defining the syndromes of infantile autism by Kanner, Bradley, Bender, Heller, De Sanctis, Weygandt, Despert, Creak and others, while the psychoanalysts Mahler, Klein, Isaacs, Rodrigué, Bettelheim and Tustin have made significant contributions to its psychological structure and its origins.

It is apparent, when reviewing the literature, that the cases described, analysed, and treated by differing therapeutic methods, with varying results, are difficult to evaluate because diagnoses are mostly insufficiently specific and the prognosis consequently uncertain. Creak tried to resolve the problem by isolating nine characteristics and specifying that to make a diagnosis of autism a child must show a specified number of them. Her method aimed at defining objective criteria, but the way in which they were interpreted by clinicians showed that they were unreliable so, if the characteristics can be interpreted so differently, it is doubtful whether her own achievement can be assessed as objective either.

Definition of Infantile Autism

In 1958 Antony organized essential data and succeeded in grouping the various syndromes in a useful and workable way as follows:—

* Previously published as 'Une théorie de l'autisme infantile' in *La psychiatrie de l'enfant*. 8. 1965. Considerable alterations have been made.

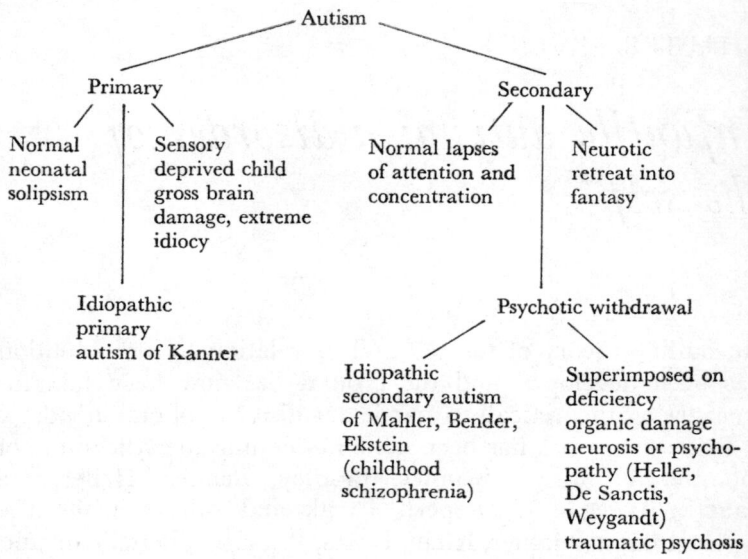

Influenced by psychoanalytic theory and Piaget's formulations as well, he related primary and secondary autism to primary and secondary narcissism.

The classification is helpful as it places the disorders in context; on the one hand the pathological forms are related to normal states, and on the other to neurosis and organic brain disease. Antony manages the variety of syndromes observed in clinical practice by claiming that each entity can combine with another, so that the cases present a continuous spectrum rather than a number of discrete disease entities.

The distinction between primary and secondary autism has been accepted by both Mahler and Tustin who have each developed it fruitfully, and they confirm Antony's view, as I do also, that there are many cases that do not fit easily to either type of disorder.

The differential diagnoses of idiopathic primary autism are between brain damage and mental defect. The less serious secondary autism is to be differentiated from the obsessional disorders though this idea has recently been contested by Meltzer: following Bion he has explored the possibility that obsessional states are more like autism than other disorders, and that the two may be genetically related.

Prognosis

Mutism is the best indication of a poor prognosis. Those children who never speak or use only a few words are less likely to recover than those who start to speak and then regress in response to a specific external event, such as the birth of a sibling, which acts traumatically (compare cases James and Anthony infra). The symptom suggests that the core of the disorder stems from the early life of the infant.

Influence of Mother

As to the influence of the mother, Antony finds, in agreement with others such as Mahler (1969), that in the primary group she is less significant than in the secondary group and that, in most cases, the influence of the mother, though always significant, is not decisive. It is on this ground that the designation of idiopathic infantile autism can be justified.

Neither Winnicott nor Bettelheim (1967), who has unique experience in this field, are at all of this opinion: Winnicott considers that there has been an environmental defect, while Bettelheim goes so far as to contend that autistic children are autistic because they came into the world and were confronted with mothers who wished for their death.

Scope and method of Present Thesis

In this paper I shall define the characteristic features of idiopathic autism and, to do this, structural models relevant to analytic procedures will be used to organize observations from cases on which I have reported in Part Three infra. Experience has also been gained through observations on other children seen for consultation and who were educable.

For present purposes it is first proposed to consider the children alone, as if the parents or other persons in the environment were non-existent. Justification for this procedure is evidently called for, especially as environmental factors were without doubt also important in both the genesis and maintenance of their disorders. The first justification is empirical: interesting observations can be made using analytic procedures, which show how influence can be exerted and changes observed in the child himself. The second justification is theoretical: it rests on the theory of the self as I have elaborated it in the earlier chapters of this book and elsewhere.

Genetic Theories

There are two groups of genetic hypotheses available:

1. Those that postulate a barrier that is set up between the child and the external world and that protects his inner world (Antony, 1958). This hypothesis presupposes that the child is born with a constitutional stimulus barrier, which is either strong or extra sensitive and becomes pathological as a defence against excessive, insufficiently reliable, or grossly defective maternal care.

2. Those that do not presuppose a barrier from the beginning, though it can and does become established later.

Mahler (1969) holds that the disorders stem from two stages of infant development that have not been outgrown. In one the infant shows primary autism and has no awareness of his self as distinct from the inanimate environment. She next distinguishes a stage in which there is a 'mother–child unity, which is characterized by delusional, omnipotent symbiotic fusion with the need-satisfying object' (ibid, p. 338). This formulation presupposes that there are two separate persons, mother and infant, who fuse. The two stages are conceived to lie at the root of two kinds of psychosis: primary autistic psychosis and symbiotic psychosis. The latter shows the characteristic 'rage–panic reactions' to minimal frustrations. Here a rudimentary and insecure boundary between the mother and infant must be assumed. These two syndromes are not incompatible, nor need they be rigidly separated; indeed, in any case under treatment, she, in line with others, holds that characteristics of each may be found and so the concept of a barrier can be used to explain some of the behaviour in the whole group and even in those children whose disorder must have crystallized in the first weeks of extrauterine life.

As to how the barrier comes into being: there are those who think that it is wholly due to environmental failure (Winnicott), or to a death wish on the part of the mother (Bettelheim); those who contend that it develops out of an infantile psychotic depression (Tustin); those who look for organic failure of the arousal mechanisms in the centrencephalic system (Rimland); finally, the origin is placed in some disorder of intrauterine life (Bender).

Relation to the 'External' Object

It is clear that the child's relation to the 'external' object must be the main focus of attention .If the views of Mahler (and others as well) are correct, there cannot be any firm distinction between what is internal and external until the child has reached a stage at which the ego is strong enough to make such distinctions; that is, until primary autism and the state of fusion have been lived through and superseded.

The idea that the relation to the 'external' object is the most elementary of all the characteristics of autism so far considered is supported by some mothers who can look back and detect that the disorder originated from soon after birth when breast-feeding had been established. If the hypothesis of such an early origin be established then it is most unlikely that the core of the disorder can be understood in terms of the child's retreat into an inner world.

(Here a difficulty in terminology arises in that what looks to the adult like 'internal' and 'external' experience of the infant or child is not so experienced by him, so I propose to put the two words in quotation marks unless the data provided by the child clearly indicates that the experience is related to a known boundary between the child's inner and outer object.)

The autistic child's relation to objects has been extensively studied. It has been observed that any object that engages the child's interest must comply with what he wants to do with it: the object can be anything from a toy to a part of a person—his hand or arm, for instance—which the child will manipulate to his own ends. If the object does not comply with the child's needs, he will either cease to be interested and treat it as if it does not exist or he will fly into a rage or panic. The objects that are used and that comply with the child's needs are called autistic or, as I would prefer, self-objects.

There is, however, another kind of relation to objects that has not received the same attention, the child's close inspection of reality. That this is possible for autistic children came as a surprise to me. When I first made the observation many years ago, it was then currently held that these children lived in an 'inner' world, and that the 'external' objects were of no interest to them except in so far as they impinged on them. A very different state of affairs has, however, been described by others besides myself and is a prominent part of Kanner's description Diatkine (1960) even goes so far as to say of one child: 'He lived in a perfectly perceived world, but one as devoid of meaning as an abstract painting composed without inspiration (p. 545). Perhaps because of its apparent meaninglessness, this 'perfectly perceived world' has been little investigated.

For many months James, who will be described in detail in Part III of this book, made pictures. The large majority of them depicted some object in the 'external' world. Among these were clocks, each of which referred to specific ones known to exist either at home or in the clinic; they were easy to recognize as reproductions though usually drawn in colour. In one picture however, there appeared numbers on the clock-dial that were unusual, and I thought they might lead to an 'inner'-world fantasy. They were the numbers on my own watch, which I had not thought he could have observed since most of the time it was covered by my jacket. He must have observed them without my noticing and then accurately recorded them in his picture.

While James's behaviour indicated the operation of quite complex structures, such as memory and the technical manipulation of objects, the lack of symbolic representation strongly suggested that he was exhibiting behaviour controlled by a state in which the 'external' object was needed to comply exactly with his requirement, which in this case means it was needed for documentation.

Allied to 'perfect perception' may be the need to keep the environment the same, for radical alterations can be disastrous; hence considerable effort may be directed towards maintaining the status quo.

James regularly put some objects in a drawer, locked it and put the key in the cupboard before leaving the room at the end of his interview. Next time he would look in the cupboard, find the key, unlock the drawer and use the objects he had put there. One day the key had disappeared. He showed no affective response; he simply occupied himself with other subjects. Later he discovered the key and unlocked the drawer—but he did not use the drawer as a place to keep objects in any more. Thus it does not seem that he recovered the key so that he could once again use the drawer, but rather to put it back where it belonged. While this might be thought of as reparative activity found in the depressive position, and this may even have been so, yet it is characteristic that the affective significance belonging to that stage in development is lacking because it is directed towards maintaining environmental stability.

Sometimes, however, the objects observed can be related to the child's behaviour. This was so in James's case for he showed detailed, apparently meaningless, interest in objects that, both at home and in the clinic, he examined very exactly. At first sight his pictures of clocks seemed to demonstrate 'perfect perception' only. He came, however, with great regularity, always arriving and leaving exactly on time, never allowing his parents to be late, as if he were ruled by a clock. Now if he had experienced his regularity 'internally', it might be expected that the 'inner clock' he seemed to possess would be expressed through 'inner', i.e. symbolic, fantasy and we might hope to and evidence of this in his drawings—but there was none. Thus James's interest in clocks, which he also took to pieces, seemed essentially part of his accurate time-keeping and could not be shought to symbolize it, though to me, as observer, it appeared fit though there was an 'internal' as well as an 'external' clock. There was, however, no evidence that he related the two; indeed, it is rather as if he himself were the clock. If this is so, then his activities reveal a self-object masked as the 'external' object.

In this discussion may be included the importance of environmental stability. James disintegrated when the treatment-room was engaged at a time when his interview should have begun; his trust and reliance on me (and so on himself also) had received a mortal blow, something disastrous had taken place. James's need for stability also transferred itself to time: it became necessary for me to be ready on time and he left immediately my watch indicated that the end of his interview had been reached.

Passive Compliance

Another prominent feature of object-relations expressed in the behaviour of autistic children is their passive compliance, which refers to the way in which they respond to intervention by an adult. If they are occupied in some activity and are wanted to do something else, it is only necessary to take the child's hand—he will then do what the adult wants passively, plastically, without any protest or any indication as to his own wishes. In a similar way, when he aims to use part of a person or an object for his own purpose, should that object not fit in with his scheme of activities, he simply desists. There is no indication that fear, disappointment, or rage lie behind this behaviour: indeed, it is only when the child begins to improve that rages and outbursts of temper take place—the very opposite of passive compliance.

Hierarchical Organization of Psychic Structures

In stating that the self-object is basic to infantile autism, it may seem that evidence of organization is being ignored. This would indeed be absurd: it is easy to notice structured behaviour in all cases.

Soon after coming to see me, James wrenched various objects out of a doll's house. Just before he left the room he replaced all of them (so I thought) but two days later, when he returned, he went straight to the box of bricks where the toys had been placed, found the toy fireplace belonging to the doll's house and promptly replaced it. In this example there is clear evidence of an ego operating, but not of symbolic representation.

It looks as if this represents an attack on his mother's body and its contents, followed by reparative activity. Examples of such behaviour can be found; indeed, facets of the mother–child relationship can be observed in all cases, and oedipal conflicts as well. For instance, masturbation may be patterned on the primal scene in which the child identifies in a delusional way with his father in genital intercourse. Interpretation of this can lead to agreement and increased activity. But these maturational patterns do not lead to development, they do not become sufficiently symbolized, and do not seem to be integrated into the self as a whole, so that the development that might be expected does not occur. It can only be concluded that the patterns of a developing hierarchy can be observed, but a hierarchy that is unorganized, disorganized, dislocated or split up. It seems that this state of affairs may be closely related to the body-image which, many observers have claimed, does not become organized for more than short periods. Acts are therefore dissociated, and compulsive repetitive behaviour takes place that does not integrate, even though the meaning is theoretically understandable.

Within the complex disorganized hierarchy it is also possible to discover split-off or unintegrated 'internal' objects. For instance, John, who chewed up objects, toys, rugs, and pieces of stuff, would in a sort of paroxysm of excitement, open his mouth and struggle with 'his' impulse to nail on to a part of my body; his arms would become raised and twitch, his fingers flexed like claws that threatened to bury themselves in my flesh. This paroxysm could be handled and partially resolved only by recognizing that his mouth and limbs did not belong to him; they were experienced as objects in their own right and separate from his rudimentary feeling of self. Interpretations framed in this way were effective in reducing anxiety and increasing control over the impulses. If the personal pronoun were used they had no effect.

My intention in presenting these examples is to suggest that if autistic children live in an 'inner' world it is not by any means felt so to be—rather they live with a world of objects (and this includes parts of their own bodies) whose arrangement is often very precise and organized, though not distributed in terms of what is inner or outer. On the basis of observations such as these it seems probable that the hypothesis of a barrier protecting an inner world is simply an assumption made by adults to explain the child's inaccessibility; this is often felt by the parent as a barrier when, in terms of the child's experience, no such feeling is established because the barrier is set up not against them but against not-self-objects. He may know and feel a barrier but it is not a defence to protect an internal object.

In the most ill children the arrangement of objects is important, but failure of these objects to comply with what will later be understood, felt or thought of as the child's requirements, does not lead to noticeable disturbances such as rage. Rage only appears as he is getting well and then it is evoked when the object does not comply with the self-object requirements.

The data are different in those children who develop very

elaborate but secondary fantasy systems which may become organized into systematic unreal world systems. In these less ill children what we call symbolic representation has taken place (Alan in Part Three). The child's object-relation systems are well developed, while observation of real objects is not nearly so detailed or precise and, indeed, is far more clearly determined by affective processes. In these cases it is possible to obtain evidence that the system is based on a self-representation (Alan, p. 204 ff). If such a system is in operation, the child either will not or cannot comply with what is required of him unless the adult enters into his world system and functions as one of the persons (objects) in it. In other words, the adult has to provide conditions under which part of the child's self can recognize the existence of the adult and fuse with him.

Finally, because it is so often overlooked, we need to recognize that near-normal bits of behaviour are also in evidence that can be of importance therapeutically. For example, when James played 'hide and seek' he was alive, excited and showed enjoyment. It developed into playing subtle tricks on me and on his mother, burlesquing and ridiculing her requests for him to do something for her.

In another case of idiopathic autism a child would behave as follows, but only at the end of an interview. When he had not got some libidinal gratification, or when he had devised some plan which he had not been able to implement during the interview, he would slip away, if my attention was not directed towards him, into another room in the clinic and place himself behind a table or chair with an escape route. This would happen particularly if he had not dared to 'rob' me of an object that he knew I kept in one of my pockets. It would be possible for him to end the interview only if some familiar object was 'stolen'— after a time he would 'steal' a familiar object from the other room and then return to his mother.

Negative Hallucination

It may sometimes be that the development of the strikingly acute capacity for observation of the object is essentially defensive. It is designed to detect even the slightest departure from known behaviour, because any alteration is terrifying.

The theory upon which this concept rests presupposes rather

complex processes in the infant. It must be said here that, as more and more is known about infant behaviour as it is directly observed, and as the analysis of adults and children becomes progressively more accurate, it seems more evident that psychosomatic events in infants are complex rather than simple. It does not therefore appear that the thesis to be elaborated, which is derived from the work of Melanie Klein, can be rejected on the basis of its complexity only.

It is assumed that from very early on the infant tends to eject violent affects into the environment, in the first place at his mother, and to record libidinal satisfactions within himself, which are then idealized as blissful. Rodrigué (1955), who worked out this thesis in greatest detail, attributed the aesthetic and gifted characteristics frequently to be observed in autistic children to the existence of this idealized object—the breast.

The idealized 'internal' object, by possessing the characteristics of omnipotence, is invulnerable to the destructive drives ejected into the external world. As a result the infant lives in a potentially terrifying world against which autistic defences are erected.

Projection is one method of reinforcing the defences that preserve the good object but at the same time increase the bad anxiety-provoking objects in the 'external' environment. If this thesis were true, one would expect the most ill children to show evidence of more or less continuous terror. This is not so, and it is necessary to assume that the terrifying destructive objects have somehow been dealt with. Rodrigué proposes and gives some evidence for his idea that the 'bad' object has been dealt with by negative hallucination: that is, it is actively removed from relation to the ego by massive denial. A triple process is thus involved in the autistic system; (a) projection, (b) a negative hallucination that eliminates the projection, (c) idealization of the 'internal' object.

This idea originated from Freud. He meant that the object, though in reality it continues to be there, is made non-existent by affective processes which, ideally speaking, prevent it from having any effect on the ego.

It is not difficult to observe the three components at work in cases under analysis, whether the patient is clinically psychotic or no. It is reflected with less pathological intensity in many adults in regression.

To gain access to the data on which the idea of negative hallucination is built, consider the frequency with which children paint a picture only to cover it with paint (most often black) so that nothing other than a black surface can be seen, and the whole picture itself is done away with because it has provoked anxiety by being a bad picture in one way or another, not well enough painted, nasty or horrifying.

This process can be observed with greater intensity of affect in autistic children. At one period in his development Anthony (p. 166) started to develop panics, for no apparent reason unless it be assumed that he had hallucinations. At these times he would switch on the electric light, though it was daylight anyway, and then his fear would disappear. At this time he also painted terrifying figures that he would cover with black paint, tear up and throw away. He was also being very destructive in other ways; he burnt the dress of a doll, he attacked a baby doll and threw it out of the window.

On the basis of Rodrigué's theory, the acute observation of reality could be conceived as a continuous scrutiny of the object lest the above defences fail at any point.

Rodrigué's case did not show the rather remarkable 'normal' early history; rather there were clear indications of feeding difficulties, which in our view only occur if the infant has progressed to the stage of the omnipotence of the object and to a degree of ego-development that renders frustration by an object possible. In short, his case suggests that he was dealing with a symbiotic psychosis in Mahler's sense and not with primary autism.

Infantile Autism as a Disorder of the Self

I have so far paid attention to the features of autism that may be primary and will now turn to considering the theory of autism on which I have been working.

It is assumed that the essential core of autism represents in distorted form the primary integrate of infancy, and that idiopathic autism is a disordered state of integration, owing its persistence to failure of the self to deintegrate.

A healthy infant is primarily a psychosomatic unity or self, which will contribute by deintegration to all psychic structures as they differentiate in the course of growth. Child development is uneven and there are periods of instability that alternate with stable states. Less attention is usually paid to the stable ones than to those in which conflict situations or severe anxieties are prominent. Thus we hear more about birth traumata, the crises of four or five months, seven months, weaning, the struggle to get control over excreta, the conflicts of the oedipal situation and the crises of adolescence, than we do about the relatively stable intervening periods.

In satisfactory development the unstable periods correspond to periods of deintegration in which increasingly defined structures are brought into being or into new relationships with each other. In the stable periods, the new advances are integrated and brought firmly together in the service of the whole.

For instance, early deintegration makes breast-feeding possible, and round this grow the beginnings of environmental adaptation. Deintegration is conceived as an activity which differs from the release-mechanism of the ethologists in being a psychic as well as a physiological process. Being derived in essential respects from the primal self, deintegrates carry within them the attribute of wholeness and treat the 'external' object as part of that wholeness. Accordingly, if the child's mother does not match the infant's need closely, she, or any part of her not provided, is deemed by the infant not to exist. At this stage the idea of omnipotence is not yet relevant, though it is potential.

A further postulate is that all the structures developed, including the perception of real objects and so of the 'external' world, conform at first to the absolute criteria of the self, i.e. it is made up of self-objects. As the infant has in the first place no means of distinguishing a 'not-self' (such an experience depends upon the development of the ego), reality in the first place is experienced as a part of the self. This concept is like Freud's concept of primary narcissism, but differs from it in that the energy in the primal self is assumed to be neutral. It is because of this conception that we have considered those aspects of infantile autism that reveal the child's relation to the 'external' object, in order to see whether the essential core of autism may not derive from a persistent primal self.

I have challenged the barrier hypothesis on two grounds. Firstly, I had not found autistic children as inaccessible as the theory would require; secondly, the idea of the barrier was related to a belief that autistic children developed an inner world but this did not apply to those of them whose fantasy systems were manifestly defective and who certainly had not developed much, if any, capacity for symbolization. It was thus the detailed working out of the hypothesis that impressed me as faulty and lacking clinical justification. I do not doubt the existence of a barrier, and James gave clear and repeated evidence of its existence (cf. infra, p. 257 ff).

It is with reference to children without evidence of capacity for symbolization that another hypothesis is particularly appealing: it states that there has been a basic catastrophe in the relation between the baby and the breast-mother. The catastrophe is conceived to be total and so there is little or no communication along with the feeding experience. This idea has also been developed by Bettelheim, who holds that the baby's active approaches to his mother have met with reactions based on a death wish; consequently the infant despairs, his development is prevented, he does not participate in it and can only comply, in a false, defensive way, with what his mother requires of him—presumably psychic death. In his therapy Bettelheim applied his idea with conspicuous success: he aimed, through a number of skilled therapists, at creating conditions under which there would be minimal impingement so that the autistic child could emerge out of himself, by deintegration, and develop in his own way. However peculiar this might be, the therapist behaved so as to facilitate the child's individuality. Tustin, working on similar lines, but using psychoanalytic techniques, also found it possible to establish relationships with autistic children.

Can these ideas be related to self theory? Only if there are defence systems in the self that could come into operation in response to impingements. They would have to be very powerful and focus on the noxious not-self so as to form an absolute barrier before there could be any possibility of an inner world being formed. It was here that Stein's work on the self (Stein, 1967) has been particularly useful. He postulated that the self has defence-systems designed to preserve individual identity and establish and maintain the difference between self and not-self; he drew on immunological researches, which have developed a theory that immunological reactions aimed to reject or annihilate not-self objects (bacteria, alien tissues, etc.); only objects that can be assimilated to the self further bio-chemical life processes.

Applying this idea that the self has well-organized defence systems, it becomes much easier to understand how a barrier is constructed. If, for instance, a baby is submitted to noxious stimuli of a pathogenic nature (either in utero, during or after birth) a persistent over-reaction of the defence-system may start to take place; this may become compounded with parts of the self by projective identification, so that a kind of auto-immune reaction sets in: this in particular would account for the persistence of the defence after the noxious stimulus had been withdrawn. Not-self objects then come to be felt as a danger to or even a total threat to life, and must be attacked, destroyed or their effect neutralized. The focus is therefore on the not-self and little or no inner world can develop; the self-integrate becomes rigid and persists.

Because of the persistence of the self-integrate, all later developments based on maturational pressures result not in deintegration but disintegration and the predominance of defence systems leads to the accumulation of violence and hostility, which is split off from any libidinal and loving communication with the object that may take place.

This hypothesis needs observations on the relation between mother and infant soon after birth, but skilled personnel have not yet been made available to embark on the necessary research project. It would be extremely difficult anyway, owing to the rarity of autism in children, so it is likely that only chance observations could be made. One such was described to me by Bianca Gordon, working with mothers in an obstetrics department of a hospital. Owing to a concatenation of circumstances a mother found it particularly difficult to relate to one baby of twins. The infant became shut off from her to such an extent that he was thought to be either blind or deaf, but tests were applied and both hearing and sight were found to be normal. Largely owing to the help given to the mother, she was able to grasp what was going on, and the subjective reasons for her inability to contact her baby. She was able to change her attitude and rescue her baby, whose subsequent development was normal. Perhaps the baby would never have become autistic, but this example does indicate how radical, and in a sense adapted, an infant's defence-reactions can be. A comparable though less successful rescue-operation is recorded in the case of Anthony (infra): the mother hated her baby at first, recognized her death wish towards it and this paved the way for love to well up in her—was it too late?

The difficulty of defining what an autistic baby looks like has made for an uncertainty that will remain until observations on such infants can be collected; but another source of information is available. However unreliable a history constructed by a mother may be, the feeding patterns recorded by some are suggestive. They state that their baby gave no trouble, was the easiest of all their babies and so forth. If, however, this statement can be gone into, it may be found that this ease in feeding is an early manifestation of the compliance shown so clearly later on. Sometimes the mother can recognize that her infant cannot be related to her and that, apart from the physical acts involved in feeding, the infant does not develop the kind of relation with her that is usual. There is no effort to relate to her, no play, no looks, no smiles, and none of the less tangible communications with her infant that are known about but are less easy to describe. Thus though the physiological instruments necessary for feeding to proceed appear to be normal, deintegration of the psychic component of self seems not to have taken place. It seems to have become split off from the soma by the time breast-feeding begins, or else very soon after it has begun. This suggests that the organism is already damaged either before or at birth, or by the mother, who may not recognize her part in it, in such a way that a pathology of integration has been formed.

The theory of the self in infancy goes some way towards understanding more of the intractable core of idiopathic autism present in varying degrees in all cases. But what of those children who do react and can, like Rodrigué's case, and like my own case, Anthony, (cf. infra), develop rages in response to frustration or teasing, and who can develop far enough to distinguish a non-self environment that fails to respond to their omnipotent demands?

In these cases integrative pathology is not so complete. Deintegration may be assumed to have been partially successful, but has led to splitting, and in some areas ego-development has taken place through interaction between the split-off bit of the self and parts of the infant's mother (breast, eyes, mouth, etc.). It must have been sufficient for fragmentary structures to have developed early on and for secondary splitting to have occurred in the ego, so that objects can be idealized, or if ejected can act as persecutors, subsequently to be attacked and hallucinated away.

It has been noted above that even the most ill children under consideration show during treatment some features of later development, but in fragmentary form. They can, as we have recorded, engage in relatively normal play, such as hide-and-seek, and can relate to their mothers physically; they will require cuddling from them or use them as a shelter against persecutory objects; they may also show oedipal characteristics and not infrequently develop gifts and talents of a specialized kind. None of these gifts or complex behaviour patterns are, however, built into the main body of the self, which in spite of them does not develop its relation to the ego and so does not give rise to a coherent feeling of self, of continuing identity and self-esteem. It makes 'external' objects conform to itself and develops a system that treats objects and parts of the body-image as the primal self or even annihilates them. To say that parts of the infant have developed but are not used for develop-ment of the primal self means that they are dislocated. In infantile autism neither of the functions of the self operate with sufficient harmony; deintegration does not occur or only does so partially. In breast-feeding the neurophysiological apparatus may operate without its psychic counterpart, and integration has become set, rigid and therefore negative. Consequently the infant cannot organize or shut out the flood of perceptual stimuli received into the self, it fails to develop the capacity to relate as a whole to internal and external objects. As the component parts of the self in relation to the whole organism cannot develop, growth is obstructed rather than facilitated. It seems that whatever ego there is reacts by splitting, as a defence against a situation controlled by the defensively destructive integrate. The split-off ego-fragments, however, mostly develop, so that later stages, pre-oedipal and oedipal features, can be observed unintegrated and prevented from being mobilized into the whole self so as to resolve conflicts in an individual form. Instead, there is a hard core of self-integration and also split-off bits of the personality that develop in perverse ways.

PART TWO

Prefatory note

Some further explanation is required as to why I have inserted in this volume a discourse on the subject of analysis and psychotherapy, and chapters on the technique of psychotherapy. There are two reasons for them.

First, though there are good empirical grounds for thinking that both child analysis and its less elaborate, though more difficult, counterpart, psychotherapy, as an abbreviated form of analysis, are effective and valuable procedures, without a theory of the self they remain empirical exercises. It is only when it is understood that a child can be treated as an individual, separate from his parents in essential respects, that therapy becomes truly meaningful and its effectiveness can be understood. It may seem, in line with the rest of this volume, that I am leaving the influence of parents far too much out of account; so, with a view to showing how relevant a child's symptoms can be in relation to his family, I have introduced a case that illustrates this common state of affairs. I would ask readers who are engaged in discovering the effectiveness of family therapy, or who have long thought that a child acts as a carrier of family disorders, to give me the credit of knowing this! Here in this volume I am occupied in putting forward a one-sided picture of childhood, in full realization that there are family problems of which a child may be merely the indicator.

My second reason for introducing chapters on analysis and therapy (an artificial but useful distinction, as I shall hope to show) is that I hold it essential to show the methods that are used in arriving at conclusions. It is not enough to provide theory and illustrative examples: how each is developed is important and especially so because, in analytical psychology, a theory of technique is only beginning to develop.

CHAPTER EIGHT

Reflections on child analysis and therapy*

Child analysis has only just begun to engage the serious attention of analytical psychologists. I shall maintain that it can make a significant contribution to individual child therapy and to our culture as well. That it has not done so until recently, at least in respect of the Jungian framework, is curious. So I shall devote the first part of this chapter to reflections upon why this is so; in the second part I am going to review some of the discoveries and findings of play therapy that have led me to conclude that radical child analysis is possible and indeed sometimes the treatment of choice. Finally, I shall show that child analysis is not in principle different from its adult equivalent, though both technically and emotionally it is more difficult.

SECTION I

Resistances to Child Analysis

Child analysis has hung behind the analytic therapy of adults even though theory would suggest it should have forged ahead. At first it was thought to be the parents who were the cause of their children's neuroses and even psychoses: it was they who seduced, threatened, neglected or over-protected their children and caused repression. But it was not long before it was shown that the reconstructions produced by adult patients, on which this theory was based, were as much the product of infantile fantasy as accounts of the real behaviour of parents themselves.

This discovery contributed powerfully to Jung's theory of primordial images and by 1912 he had established that they

---

* Previously published as 'Riflessioni sull'analisi infantile', in *Rivista di psicologia analitica.* 4, 2. 1973. It was delivered at a conference entitled 'Jung e la cultura europea' held in Rome in the same year. Some revisions have been made.

underlie the conflicts under consideration. Then, as the result of long, intensive and wide-ranging research, he went on to formulate and develop his concept of archetypes and to postulate not the inheritance of the images themselves, but of patterns of psychic functioning analogous to instincts and having spiritual potential. The theory of the inheritance of psychic functions had important bearing on child psychology and Jung was fully aware of it. He was even led to state that 'dreams and images appear before the soul of the child, shaping his whole destiny as well as those retrospective intuitions which reach far back beyond the range of childhood experience into the life of our ancestors' (1948, p. 52) and again, 'The child's inheritance is highly differentiated and consists of mnemonic deposits accruing from all the experience of our ancestors' (ibid, p. 53).

I have discussed the validity of these statements in my book *Children as individuals* and will not repeat myself, but my object in quoting them here is to draw attention to a theoretical position that positively cries out for a thorough investigation of childhood itself and would seem also to suggest a prominent place for child analysts; it even suggests that every child might have a child analyst available just as he has a physical doctor that his parents can consult. Surely, if a child has so much psychic inheritance, his psyche must be complex, and surely there would, especially in view of the infantile roots of neuroses, be need of special help for those children who run into difficulties arising from the sheer complexity of their own psychic processes. Furthermore, it is known that the way small children experience their parents is often controlled by archetypal forms, which can make them inaccessible to their real parents; so there develops a considerable part of a child's individuation from which parents are excluded and indeed into which it is not their place to intrude.

But no analytical psychologists followed up this line until I started my own work. It may well be said that Frances Wickes studied the relation of children to their parents; but she swung away from investigating unconscious processes in childhood, partly because she was so much impressed by the importance of parental neurosis in the genesis of childhood disorders, and partly from anxiety lest the dreaded archetypes be roused from the depths and overwhelm the child's ego. Jung himself, however, had studied cases of children in some of his earlier publications: there is not only Anna to cite (Jung, 1910) but also a case of neurosis in a child of eleven in 'The theory of psycho-analysis'; in addition, there is a short study of a four-year-old boy with whom he adopted Adlerian-like methods in order to reinforce the child's ego. In 'The significance of the father in the destiny of the individual' (1949) a child is cited as an example; then there are various references to children's dreams and paintings, and finally the lengthy seminars on children's dreams which, regrettably, he never worked forward to a state in which they could be published. Thus much background work had been done before I began to investigate the un-conscious process *with* as well as *in* a child; and it took me many years to do it.

When I was starting my work I was impressed by a sort of passive but tolerant resistance on the part of colleagues, and one of my analysts thought my interest was due to my own infantile characteristics. In retrospect I can say that it was a half-truth because it did not work out quite as I or he had expected: indeed it was my resistance to treating children that was infantile, not my interest in them, for I continued to believe, when in difficulties with a child, that this was due to interference by his parents' unconscious. It took many years' work to see that, however true that might be, it was used to obscure my own technical and affective deficiencies. It was only when I could change my attitude that I saw there was a place for child therapy as a serious and valuable discipline of its own, in principle like adult analysis though, in application, significantly different.

Lawrey Hawkey (1945 and 1947) was the first to publish a detailed study in child analytic therapy from a Jungian point of view. Subsequently members of the London Society of Analytical Psychology treated children, and this work is recorded in a number of papers by Margaret Aldridge, Robert Moody, Dorothy Tate *et al.* in the *Journal of analytical psychology*, while in Switzerland there have been Jolande Jacobi and Dora Kalff (who became interested in Margaret Lowenfeld's sand-tray techniques), and also Zublin. They have, over the years, accumulated much experience, and one might have thought that they would want to pass this on by training others.

In Israel, under the aegis of Eric Neumann, a group was

formed that trained child therapists—I will return later to why this should be—but nowhere else in the world was anything comparable started till now in London; we do not yet know whether our venture will succeed. This project has a very long history, which I will not record in detail; I will only say that it was about fifteen years ago that attempts were made to form a small discussion group. It was attacked as being too exclusive and virtually broken up. The group was vulnerable because those relatively competent in the field had doubts and anxieties of the following kinds: did any of us know enough, was our knowledge sufficiently organized, were there enough people to do this training? Their worries were not helped by doubts expressed from within the general body of the Society, that training in child therapy would overstrain the resources available for training in the analysis of adults.

There were also objections not so much to therapy being done with children as to any enquiry into what was meant by therapy or into what happened when therapy was being pursued. The term *analysis* raised even greater anxieties. Looking back on it all, one cannot avoid the reflection that, if child analysis was to develop, children would get what was the prerogative of adults: *this must not happen* was implied. The struggle to get something going did at last lead to the formation of a special section in the society to study children; at first it flourished but eventually collapsed, at about the time when a project to train child analysts came into being.

This pattern of resistance is not confined to analytical psychology; it is also shown in psychoanalysis. Indeed, I have been informed that Anna Freud was compelled to start her Child Therapy Clinic and training outside the Institute of Psychoanalysis in London, and only recently has training in child psychoanalysis been generally instituted. So there seem to be objections of a similar kind among analysts of both schools, and our experience cannot be put down only to Jung's emphasis on parents as the source of infant disorders.

An argument against child analysis that helps to generalize the problem is that cases are difficult or impossible to obtain; parents cannot be induced to take their child frequently for treatment interviews and schools will not allow for the child's frequent absences. There is something to be said for both these objections, though they also apply to the analysis of adults who cannot (or protest that they cannot) get time off work, or whose internal parents raise the strongest objections to anything being done. In the case of children there are other external difficulties: many parents do not like, or even actively oppose the idea of admitting failure, whether real or imagined, often because it threatens their omnipotence or because it seems a blow to their self-esteem; they often feel that they do not want to have somebody doing something with their children that they do not understand. Again, they may feel jealous and envious that their child should benefit in a way that had not been possible for them; so they may prefer to send their child away to boarding school, or to a special school where well-understood educational methods are used with which they are or have been familiar through their own education when they also were children. In this way they capitalize on the cultural style of scepticism and they object that it is not really necessary, so that only when it is very obvious to them will they overcome their objections. All these resistances combine, even today, to make it impossible for anybody to build a child analytic practice and make a good living out of it.

This state of affairs applies, in my experience, to many analysts themselves whose children are in difficulties: they may (narcissistically) use it to further their own development and let their children go through unproductive suffering and pain or they may prefer to obtain more analytic help for themselves. But this does not always work and in the end their children grow up and ask for the analysis they might have had many years earlier. The term *narcissism* is meant descriptively and not in its pejorative sense, and I fully recognize that there is often a scientific basis for parents' desire to seek analysis because their own psychopathology is interfering with their child's mental health. The case for their so doing was well argued by Roland Cahen (1955) and replied to by myself (1957).

Through analytic experience with parents it is possible to say with some certainty that these resistances are not based on reality but are due to the fantasies of parents about their children. Thus the child that is abnormal comes to represent a part of themselves that is projected into the child; but besides this, and in the background, it is the child archetype that gives rise to anxiety, because there is no symbol through which it can become conscious. This raises the question of parents in analysis who have difficult or neurotic children. Whether the child gets help depends very much upon the attitude of the analyst: some will resist their patient's claim that their child needs the sort of help they themselves are getting, and will treat the assertion as a symptom. So indeed it may be, but it may also be true that their child does need treatment and this should be given adequate and realistic recognition.

I hope that I have said enough to show that such objections are a matter worthy of investigation in their personal and social aspects, and here I may take up the fact that the introduction of training in child therapy by analytical psychologists began in Israel, where the ties of family life were loosened and many children were brought up in kibbutzim. The consequences of this situation are complex and the need for it arose out of unusual circumstances, but it does suggest that it may have made a more objective view of children's needs possible.

In concluding the first part of this chapter I should like to meet the criticism that I am simply describing, in a particular context, difficulties and resistances that arise in the case of any new venture. If that is the impression I have given, then I have not conveyed what I mean. It is true that any new departure will arouse objections that have to be met squarely before one can go forward; but in the case of children a special tendency to concretism comes into play, and the fact that it concerns children raises more affect. For example, once you start talking effectively about children to a group, it is usual for at least one member to express emotion; this is required because everybody's unconscious is touched but most people decide not to show it, so there has to be a safety valve. In this respect the subject of child analysis is different from any other.

There may be another reason for marking these objections out for special attention. In his paper on 'The child archetype' Jung considered the conflicts that arise over a new under-taking, and he sets out stages in the recognition of the child archetype as being especially related to realization of the self. The first stage is that of the misunderstood and unjustly treated child with overweaning pretentions; the next is that of inflation through idealization of the child as hero. Finally, unconscious fantasy becomes objectified and this leads on to the shift in the centre of the person from ego to self. The subject of child analysis and therapy gains especial importance from this consideration: the tendency to reject child analysis and blame parents belongs to the first stage, and is the one I have especially considered here. Idealization of the child leads to the second stage. This is found among child therapists who claim that it does not matter what the parents are really like, the child can get on well in spite of them. Stage three suggests a more realistic assessment of the child's capacity and relation to parents and analyst.

Jung's essay on the child archetype is about individuation, which he always links with the history of culture. In *Children as individuals* I considered the specific role of the child in the individuation of parents, and have also related the family to cultural influences. It was with these ideas in mind that I thought it worth looking at the conflicts surrounding child analysis, to see whether they reflected stages in the individuation process. That they seem to do so gives this chapter special relevance to the theme of this book.

Child Therapy and Child Analysis

Children's dreams and fantasies evoked fascination and considerable scientific interest in Jung; but, like Frances Wickes, he was concerned lest analysis of children should push them back among the archetypes at a time in their lives when they need to emerge from them. So in considering child analysis, if it is to be more than an academic exercise, it must be shown that it is felt as valuable by the child himself and that it has therapeutic effects. I now wish to consider the work of a number of Jungian child therapists, especially those practising on their own in Switzerland and Italy; maybe there are others and in some other countries as well—but these are the ones that I know of from personal experience. It is to be regretted that only Dora Kalff, Jolande Jacobi and Zublin have published their findings.

As far as I understand it, the idea they work on, though this is of course not all that they do, is one that has entered into my own investigations. They give children increased opportunity to form their fantasies by making pictures or through modelling in various materials. Dora Kalff, as I have already remarked, has used Lowenfeld's sand-tray technique, in which a large selection of toys are available to help the children in self-expression. She became especially interested in the occurrence of mandala-like patterns.

By and large I believe all these approaches may be classed as play techniques, but ones that lay special importance on archetypal forms. Now the results show, as my own did too, that giving form to archetypal elements helps rather than hinders child development. And there are sometimes clear indications that the value children gain is not so different from that experienced by adults. It may therefore be concluded that in childhood the archetypes play a role closely analogous to that found in adults, if not essentially the same.

I may instance in this connection the capacity of some children to use magical procedures. It is most interesting: they feel 'instinctively' that a magic circle expresses a system that protects something valuable in themselves against dangerous attacks (real or imagined) coming from outside; or they may feel that if they put a bad object inside the circle they will keep it under control for the time being. Again the valuable thing inside may be a self-representation, neither good nor bad.

By using play, opportunities are given for self-expression but in, it must be added, a safe and reliable environment with a person—a therapist—there. He may not say anything about archetypes to the child, he may indeed ingenuously deny any influence at all in producing them. You will not be deceived; a therapist's attitude cannot be hidden and he will betray it in many indirect ways: by providing paper and paints, or by appreciating some pictures or sand-tray patterns more than others. It is absolutely impossible to conceal such attitudes from a child and, whether you like it or not, the production of archetypal pictures will be facilitated by the adult's sympathetic valuing attitude. The attitude is needed and should not be denied, for where it is absent the child will conceal his inner life from the adult.

I would remind you here that in his childhood Jung carved a manikin from the end of a ruler, made a bed for it in his pencil-case, where he also placed a stone, and hid it up in the attic where he knew nobody would go: 'I knew', he writes, 'that not a soul would ever find it there. No one could discover my secret and destroy it' (1963, p. 34). This illustrates the lengths to which a child can go when his inner being faces real or imagined incompatible, wrong, or damaging attitudes of adults.

Though all this evidence is not derived from the analysis of children, as I understand it, yet it is encouraging; it suggests that the archetypes are not something that are dangerous to many children and that on the contrary they underlie ego-processes and, far from needing to be avoided, they are fruitful sources of growth.

But do children themselves find that going to a therapist is valuable? There can be no doubt about it, for they want to come for it even if they only sometimes say so in words; they will regret it when the sessions have to stop and when they no longer feel the need of them they will recognize it and voluntarily end their treatment, much as an adult will do.

A feature of childhood is the great maturational potential to be found there, by which I mean the child's inherent capacity for growth, mental as well as physical. All aspects of the child are involved, conscious and unconscious, and this is expressed in numerous and varied ways. Changes take place in the archetypal forms: in the libido, which moves through stages in its development from the oral via the anal to genital organization, and in the ego, which becomes progressively stronger; together they ensure that new experiences are being almost continually organized into the self. This goes on whether a child is mentally healthy or disordered, whether the parents are good enough, or whether the family falls below the level in which a child can possibly be healthy. Thus, in very unhealthy children, even in the most severe cases of infantile autism, who are disturbed from birth and probably before, there is evidence of libidinal growth and of organized perception of reality.

For maturation to proceed evenly there needs to be what has been appropriately called by D. Winnicott a 'facilitating environment'. In normal conditions this is provided by the family, the school and all the increasing number of those who assist parents in bringing up their children. Then there are those more especially concerned with maturation and its disorders; the child therapists. Non-Jungian ones are fairly numerous, they provide help of various kinds; they are a special aspect and form of the facilitating environment and their interest in the child's inner world gives an opportunity to bring out into the open, and into relation with another person, what he has felt it necessary to conceal. Once this has happened maturation can often take over and the concealed part becomes reorganized in the self, taking in new and adapted forms useful in everyday living. Thus they produce therapeutic effects, often explicitly though more often implicitly, appreciated by the children themselves.

There are many other ways in which therapy can take place. For a long time it has been known that if parents and children visit a psychiatrist or a team, such as that provided in child guidance clinics, rather quick results are sometimes obtained for which little more than theoretical speculations or the generalized idea of maturation can be offered as causes. Recently, however, a number of techniques have been developed that elucidate this phenomena. Perhaps the most enlightening has been the work of Winnicott (1971), whose capacity to let a child form a relationship of trust was unusual, so that in a single interview the conflict in the child became clear and its resolution could begin. He communicated the content of the situation to the parents and so the family continued to facilitate the child's recovery. Some of the children who were treated in this way were seriously disturbed; even they made quite good recoveries, but I must emphasize that the techniques he used were based on personal qualities of long experience and training in psychoanalysis. They require these prerequisites and cannot be repeated without them.

These ways of helping children and families have recently been supplemented by family interviews in which patterns of interaction to an interview situation bring to light the patterns of family life and, among other things, go far to show up who is the patient if there be one only or who are the patients if there are several. By this method also rather dramatic results can sometimes be achieved. In spite of the good results from these methods, it should be borne in mind that there is danger in relying upon a child's maturational potential. It may lead to the basic conflict being covered over successfully for quite a long time, and when it does re-emerge it may be more difficult to analyse.

What is meant by child analysis, and what is the difference between therapy and analysis? It is partly (1) a matter of how much a child needs of a special situation and partly (2) a matter of the technique used.

Indications for Child Analysis

To grasp how much time and skill a child needs, it is necessary to understand how the need for analysis arises and so to know more about child development. The idea that Jung adhered to in the case of adults can be applied to children: the archetypes form the basis for maturation and out of their impact with the environment ego-fragments form and then coalesce to make a central ego-nucleus. If parents unwittingly interfere in this process and the effects are noted, then a change in their attitudes will be enough for the growth processes to right themselves more or less automatically.

This formulation applies quite well to a number of situations, but anybody working for long in child therapy will come across its limitations:

1. Parents may undergo successful analytic treatment, but the child remains the same as before.
2. Parents may refuse therapy on the grounds that they do not need it.
3. However much they are treated, parents cannot do enough with themselves to help their children sufficiently, or what they have done does not cure them. Perhaps this is best expressed in the case of children of analysts or of parents who have been analysed.

These cases suggest there is room for considering what more can be done for the children. In the first case, the child seems to be in difficulties in his own right, for the removal of the parents' bad influence is not enough and so either the child has run into difficulties on his own, or else he has encapsulated the bad part of the parents within himself and this does not change when the parents do. In the second case, it may or may not be so; in the third, the well-intentioned parents cannot change the child, who needs help because his conflicts have not originated in his parents at all.

Another way of approaching the problem is to study the child's history as recounted by the parents, even though such histories may not be very reliable in detail and may even be grossly at fault, because guilt or other complicating emotions make the parents give wrong emphasis and distort facts. In spite of these defects, if the history gives clear evidence of disturbance before the age of two, then it is unlikely that treating the parents will be sufficient. This observation raises the subject of the mother–infant relation.

Right from the start, the mother-infant set-up is two-sided and is best thought of in this light. In extreme cases, whatever a mother does, her baby will not thrive. Of course that situation is rare, and is mostly due to a mother not understanding or not being able to meet her baby's needs. The mother's resources may be depleted, so that the mother–infant couple cannot get along together and the baby will suffer more or less seriously. Even then recovery may take place, but also it may not.

I do not want it to be thought that all severe children's disorders begin in infancy, but a bad start from which recovery does not take place is difficult and ultimately impossible to redress completely; there will at best always be a scar. There are many comparable situations that arise all along the line as a child grows up, and if there is a bad start these are more likely to repeat and so become part of the child-self not accessible to parents.

Child Analysis

I hope this brief statement will give some indications of the problems that confront a child therapist and that he has to consider when deciding whether analysis is indicated or not.

You may think that I have not said enough about the family, but the importance of parents, who usually contribute so much to the cause of disorders in childhood, is well established; and it is also well known that if the damage is sufficiently recent, or takes place at the level of identification, changes in parents will lead to corresponding alterations in the child. In this case the treatment of the parents alone will be sufficient because they alone are the patients.

In the field of child psychiatry the difficulty in deciding who is the patient has led to recurrent swings between focusing on either a child or his parents. There is at present a swing back to investigating the family as a whole, which is called 'family therapy'. It is understandable, in view of the difficulties in sorting out causes and what can be done about them, that a relatively one-eyed or simple approach or theory should be adopted. It may have the aim of producing quicker or better results or, in the case of family therapy, it may be held that to improve personal relations as a whole will be prophylactic. These are worthy aims and can be criticized only if they are used to obscure the reality that many children are not cured by changes in their environment, though they may seem better for the time being. The other point of view, that if a child appears ill then he needs treatment quite apart from the state of the family in which he lives, is an equally simplistic conception. It is still held by some child therapists and it is equally one-eyed.

I think I have said enough to conclude that there exist children who show clear evidence of intrapsychic damage of long standing, and whose defences are so strong that they cannot be easily modified because of the very intense and primitive affects that are lurking in the background. If these children are removed from the home environment, or if treatments are used that aim to rely on stimulating or freeing the maturation potential, then, in each case, there is a risk of short-term improvement, which results in a pseudo-maturity rather than genuine growth and which leaves the underlying condition unchanged but masked. To minimize these risks child analysis is indicated, and I will now discuss what this means in contrast to shorter therapies.

The aim of child analysis is to provide a special situation in which disturbances buried beneath complex defences can be reached. The early situation may be one in which play with toys has not been achieved and it is perhaps before the period in which the child has much capacity to use paints, pencil and paper. Therefore, he will need to make at some time a very primitive relation to his analyst, in which play materials need not be emphasized. Usually a few are then sufficient for the child's purpose, though he may bring his own toys if he feels inclined to supplement the ones he is given; these are put in a special place, usually a cupboard or drawer, to which nobody but he has access.

The selection of toys can be facilitated by a discussion with parents, who will tell you that there are a lot of neglected toys lying in the play cupboard, or that there are some their child has liked for a long time. It is these that need to be provided in addition to the ones he may bring along; they may be added to his basic collection or taken away again. There is room for personal variation here because analysts differ in what they prefer and are comfortable with, in the different conditions that may arise.

During his three years' analysis, a boy of eight regularly used the following toys:

1. Paper from a fairly large drawing and painting book. The paper was used for drawing on, making darts and a number of special constructional activities.
2. Chalks and a pencil.
3. Scissors.
4. A small box of 'Lego' i.e., interlocking bricks.
5. A toy gun with bullets.
6. Small plastic figures of human beings.
7. A model petrol station (its box proved useful as a background for shooting).
8. A small collection of plastic animals (not much used).
9. A collection of six Matchbox motor cars.
10. Many objects in my room: ornaments, jars, cushions, books, etc.
11. My body: mouth and belly most of all.

From time to time he brought additional toys, varying from a huge soft doll, as big as or bigger than a baby, to electronic equipment. At the end of his analysis he took with him the chalks, the box of bricks, the toy gun, the plastic figures, the model petrol station, the plastic animals and the Matchbox motor cars.

I saw him in my ordinary consulting-room in which I see adults, and he came five times a week. This gives you a sample of the physical conditions provided. I am often asked about them and I think this is a fair picture, but with a smaller child a play-room makes it easier to cope with those activities that are not easy for the child to control and which can lead to considerable disorder and mess.

The main part of child analysis proper is not, however, the use of toys; it consists in the analyst's verbalizing and interpreting what is going on and urging the child to do likewise. The object of using interpretation is the same as in adult analysis, to bring unconscious contents into consciousness and to help the child in controlling anxiety; it is, I hope, self-evident that the analyst will need to couch his communications in language that the child can appreciate, so that intellectual formulations in particular are seldom used.

In child analyses also the transference/countertransference set-up becomes central. It is necessary to rely on it because it provides the main matter for analysis. The child's communication, whether it is in play or words, always contains a reference to his analyst. All of it is a communication to somebody, the analyst as parent, teacher, brother or sister, or the analyst as a construct of his imagination, an archetypal form; or it may be only a statement that he wishes or needs to be left alone. A specially important feature during regression is the transference to the analyst's communications as a whole: they may become a noise, something to be tolerated, a sort of magic, a source of confusion, or an unwarranted intrusion and so on. All this can be observed in adult analyses as well, but with children it is very important for the analyst to recognize quickly what is happening so that he can deal with it as soon as possible.

The counter-transference is more important than in adult analysis because of the greater affective liveliness of a real child, which hits the analyst's unconscious and constellates the child archetype. In his essay 'The child archetype', Jung summarizes typical attitudes towards it which I have already referred to earlier in this chapter, though in a different context, and which I now want to consider in rather more detail.

(a) He says: 'The initial stage [of] personal infantilism presents the picture of an "abandoned" or misunderstood and unjustly treated child with overweening pretentions'.

One of the commonest features among child therapists is the tendency to identify with the child because of his seemingly impossible position; and they feel that if therapy is not progressing it is, as I said earlier on, the parents' fault; this attitude can even make the progress of analysis almost impossible. I do not refer so much to cases where it is really true, as when it obscures the transference content of the child's communication.

(b) The second stage is that of inflation. The child hero is idealized as a compensation for a sense of inferiority. In this stage, Jung says, the problem is to identify fantasies and so to distinguish the real from the imagined parents and recognize that it is not the parents who are at fault.

(c) The third stage distinguished by Jung is the developing

relationship to the child archetype, which can then be understood as a self-symbol: this corresponds to recognition of real children as people, individuals in their own right even in their earliest formative periods. Mothers could have told us about this long, long ago, and children as well for that matter, if we could have listened and noticed: for Jungian analysts this understanding has come about after a long, roundabout journey, going step by step through the surrounding environment, through the superficial network of diversions until finally they have discovered the central individuality of the child.

To illustrate these ideas from analytic practice: the child I have referred to, when aged eleven and in the third year of his analysis, talked about his parents as follows: he referred to his mother as quite mad and even gave precise details about her emotionality and disorganized thinking. He also referred to his father as a piece of furniture in the house, ending up with 'If the house went up in flames he would go with it.'

He values his analysis very highly: I am the only person who understands him, he says, and the only person that cares for him; he could not do without me. These statements are seductive, especially as I knew that his father was a precariously compensated manic-depressive and had been in analysis for many years; recently he had broken down and had become quite severely depressed. His mother, also in analysis, was in reality a very disorganized person and at times incapable of understanding her child. She claimed to know about him intuitively, but this was often a mask for a projection that sometimes reached delusional proportions.

There was thus much that could give rise to a countertransference corresponding to the first described above. In that case I should have concluded that the child was only making an objectively true statement and I might have overlooked his pretensions, of which there were many. Each of his statements about his parents, however, could also be related to bits of my behaviour, for when he talked about his mother he was also referring to his feeling about some of the things I said to him; when he referred to his father he also referred to the way I sat in my chair and did not play with him. Interpreting the transference in each of these situations became essential if analysis was to proceed. By doing so a situation was created in which he could analyse his own feelings, thoughts and affects, and then he could discover that I am different from his parents, and in which ways, and so he could reach the projections he made on to them and on to others; it was also possible to sort out what comes from introjection of his parents and what is part of himself. In arriving at these conclusions it was necessary to discriminate interpretations made upon the objective and the subjective planes which, as Jung found, lead to further understanding and realization of the self.

When this child's idealization of me and denigration of his parents and of his schoolmasters was viewed upon the subjective plane, it was clear that this was the result of splitting his objects into good and bad ones. Seeing me as good and bad at once is a step in the direction of integration and of recognizing his parents and himself as both rather than one or the other. As a consequence of this analytic work he became easier for his parents to manage, and he did not constellate their psychopathology to the same extent. It was this 'improvement' that led them to end his analysis and raised the interesting and distressing question of how much health a pathological family can tolerate.

The capacity to proceed as I have described depends upon reaching stage three in Jung's scheme. Stage two—idealization of the child—would be to feel that the parents' pathology was of no consequence and that the child could himself reach mental health on his own. His pretentiousness, expressed in many ways, but especially in his view that it was absurd that he had to go to school at all—that he could learn all he needed without it, and so forth—could, under the influence of a stage two countertransference, lead the therapist to think that his was a realistic view of the matter (there was indeed much in it) and so make analysis of this state impossible. His ideas were partly supported by his parents, who could neither see nor tolerate the depression that lay behind it; his pretentions covered a deep sense of his own inadequacy, which he despaired of changing. Yet it was basically this feeling that had been crippling his capacity to organize his ideas into a form he could use at home, and that had made it largely impossible to work effectively at school.

CHAPTER NINE

Family interviews

My training in analytical psychology taught me to approach the problem of a child from without inwards. First the family needed investigation, before the problem of the child, if he had one, could be defined; in short, whether anything was wrong with him was discovered negatively. The idea behind this approach was that a child's individuality was not practically significant, and that when the disturbing factors originating in his parents were removed then their child would spontaneously recover. Today this generalization is no longer tenable, though there are children to whom it applies. In any case, it remains important to evaluate the components that enter into a child's neuroses: how much derives from his parents and how much originates in him? In this chapter I shall describe a technique that aims to elucidate this problem by interviewing as many of the family as come to see me together.

The technique can be put to a variety of uses and it cannot always be applied because a minimal style of openness between the members of a family is required. In addition there can be matters between the parents that they do not find relevant to their children and that they have deliberately hidden and wish to communicate in the child's absence. There can be no point in forcing such matters out into the open when the need for privacy is justified. Sometimes parents may have rather definite ideas about how they want the interviews arranged: they may, for instance, want to see the therapist before the child even comes for his interview. So the technique can be adapted or even not used at all. I have nonetheless found it useful in a rather wide spectrum of families.

The technique derived from working for many years in Child Guidance Clinics, in which the intake interview procedure involved a number of interviews by different specialized members of a team. The child was seen first by a psychologist for testing and would also have an interview with the psychiatrist, who would assess his emotional state; meanwhile a parent, usually the mother, would be interviewed by the psychiatric social worker, whose aim would be to discover why the child had been brought, what his symptoms were and how they had developed. If she could make an assessment of the situation at home and at school, so much the better.

In 1952 I published my view that this approach had disadvantages and suggested that the complicated transference situations that arose were obscured by splitting and could be better managed by sampling the child's relation to his parents, and their relation to him and each other, in a single stable setting; if separating the members of the family becomes desirable, it can be done later.

Since the family comes for a consultation because of a child, the parents usually want me to say something about him. So I start with a token interview with the child before seeing as many of the family as have come to the interview. Also present is the psychiatric social worker so that she can know what has gone on and be included in the treatment from the start. In addition, she can act as an observer, who forms views of her own that shed light on the proceedings, and as a screen on which projections are made; finally, she can look after the children if I am not in the room or am concentrating on their parents.

The first interview is conducted without any arrangements about who comes to it. The practice of letting it be known that all the family should come, as if this were required of them, often specially stating that the father should come, has undesirable features. The one I consider most unfortunate is that it interferes with the habitual structure of a particular family's life and may conceal the way in which responsibility for the care of children is habitually taken. I recognize that the problem is complex and that a particular father who did not come, because not asked to do so, would have come if he had been requested, but his not coming does suggest that he leaves the main responsibility to his wife, and that is significant.

I did not start off with the idea of conducting family therapy. When I saw parents and children together it was rather at first with the idea of making a provisional assessment. Over the years it appeared, however, that the interviews had therapeutic effects and that they provided the basis for short treatments; or one meeting, or a few, could take place in order to define the focus of the disorder, round which further treatment could develop if needed.

The aim is not to make a thorough diagnosis, which can be deferred, if necessary, for a later occasion—even until the end of all the interviews or of therapy; nor is it primarily to collect information. It is to create a situation that the members of a family can use for their own purposes. With these ideas in mind, I constructed a framework for the first interview. The child is first to be seen on his own and after him his parents, with or without the child present, according to the expressed wishes of the people concerned.

1. I go into the waiting-room, say that I am 'Dr. Fordham', that I should like to see the child (using his Christian name) first, and that after this I shall want to see his parents as well. Proceeding thus tests the security of the child in relation to his parents; it creates a situation of stress that is reacted to in various ways. Some children come along with me quite easily; others, after a display of anxiety, succeed in making it. Much depends on how the parent manages the situation, and useful information can be obtained by watching how the child and his parents behave—the degree of mother's narcissism, for instance, and whether her husband supports it or not. Usually, if the child shrinks back, starts to cry and his parents cannot reassure him rather easily—in short, if there is too much anxiety that cannot be managed—I ask the members of the family present to come along together into the play-room, which has comfortable chairs for the adults to sit in.

2. Supposing the child comes along alone, it is useful to observe how long it takes for him to settle down in the room to some pattern of play, drawing, talking, etc. Having received an impression of what he is like—this usually takes up to fifteen minutes, though if he starts producing his conflicts I prolong it, but I try to avoid doing so—I tell the child that it is time to fetch his parents and ask if he would like to do it. If he does not want to, or is too young to take the responsibility, then I go to bring them in myself. This is the second stress to which the child is subjected and the social worker can deal with any crisis that may arise.

Here is an example of managing a situation with manifest anxiety. John was in the waiting-room with his mother. When I announced myself he shrank against her and looked frightened. Quite firmly and kindly his mother said, 'Now go along with the doctor'. I held out my hand. With evident trepidation, he walked along with me. While we were going along together, I started to say: 'I know doctors often do things to a child that he does not ask to have done to him, so you may be imagining me to be a doctor who is going to do something to you that you do not like'. By that time we were in the play-room and he looked quite different. He agreed with enthusiasm and asserted that he hated doctors because they operated on him and stuck things into him. As he talked he pointed to his eye, which had a slight squint, meaning that a doctor wanted to operate upon him for this.

After this he turned to the toys with a feverish restless activity that made the development of a game impossible.

These observations could be made in about fifteen minutes and they were enough for me to see John's mother and have something to contribute if required. I then asked him whether he would like to fetch his mother and he scampered out of the room and brought her in. My conclusion had been:

1. John trusted his mother enough to feel that, though he was frightened, she would not play tricks on him or deceive him.
2. There were quite severe castration anxieties and a kind of restless manic defence against anxieties of a depressive kind. These might be due to regression or might be the primary root of his disorder.

I have selected this example to illustrate the immediate use of transference interpretation, which is often valuable.

When the parent or parents, and other members of the family also, as seems convenient, are in the room and everybody is seated, playing or standing about, I say something that will start the parents talking and thereafter leave the situation to develop with as little intervention as possible, the aim being to let the family reveal how its members function.

If it can be made clear that I want to know what they have to tell me and if it can also be got across that I aim to work together with the members of the family to find out more about what bothers them, then they are more likely to speak freely and give information in their own way; so I structure the interview as little as possible and in particular make no attempt to collect a history, though most parents usually reflect on how the present conditions came about. Interpretations may again facilitate working together by providing insights into what is being said or done, with a view to helping the process along.

Case One

In this case the family used the clinic quite effectively to re-establish a well-defined pattern of family life. The family needed to be treated as a unit in the sense of going beyond the individual members of it. The assumption used is that the child showed symptoms that could be taken as an indicator of the state of the family as a whole. As will be seen, it was structured round the father as the dominant member, to whom the mother was submissive. To alter this pattern in a Jewish family would be a major operation even if it had been desirable. The boy was the eldest son and his symptoms hit the family pattern hard enough for his parents to search for help so as to defend it.

James, aged two and a half, separated rather easily but in an excited way; the excitement continued throughout the interview when his parents were present. There was the tendency to switch from one subject to another.; it suggested a 'manic' basis for reaction under stress. This might be relatively unimportant or might be serious.

After a short time I fetched his parents and they settled down quickly. James's mother looked rather worn out; not so his father—a young, neatly-dressed Rabbi, who was well in charge of himself. Mother started talking, he added comments and tried to dominate the situation as the interview went on.

It was no surprise to hear that James was abnormally aggressive and mother thought he was becoming a danger to his younger brother. He was, in addition, faecally incontinent and it appeared that he had been excluded from a nursery school on account of it; on this I expressed doubts, but both parents were sure of it. Mother spoke calmly but in a depressed, monotonous, helpless voice. James had been difficult from the start: a colicky baby, who cried a lot. Mother had caught German measles when pregnant and feared she might have damaged the baby in utero.

As he grew up he started tantrums and he cried and whined if he could not get what he wanted but was very independent and would run away when in the park with his mother. Because she had his baby brother to look after, and had a prolapse of the uterus as well, she could not control him and the impression was given of her being led a terrible dance trying to catch him as he rushed away from her.

Without making his wife feel too uncomfortable, James's father started making positive remarks about his son, to complement his wife's depressed view rather than to criticize her. James was, it is true, 'never an affectionate type': he 'pushes you away', 'not affectionate, no cuddling', but except when jealous he often helped the little one; he loved music, pictures and books; he was very quick and knew all about the potty, even telling the baby what to do: it was for babies to sit on, not for him.

So as to decide about the relevance of James's restlessness I said I wanted to see James several times and then the family and I could meet again. My object was to find out how disorganized his play could be.

In my interviews with him alone the play was diffuse and restless at first, but he eventually settled down to water-play, which he stuck to; he was manageable if you were quick to help when he got into difficulties with the play-material; he accepted help over turning the tap on and off or pulling out and inserting the plug in the sink. He submitted to having the sleeves of his jersey rolled up and having a towel put round him so that he did not get too wet.

Meanwhile James's mother was being seen by the social worker, who went into her physical state. Mother did not, in fact, have a prolapse but anaemia, for which she could and did get treatment. These interviews supported the mother; the father, who came along each time as well, remained in the waiting-room looking rather left out. Neither I nor the social worker did anything about this, since he had made it abundantly clear that he was not at fault.

After several interviews with James, I thought I knew enough to review the situation: it was quite clear that he was a restless child, not too seriously disturbed in this respect, but would be hard for a depressed mother to manage. Mother and father were in the room with the social worker when I came in and sat down, hesitating before I said anything. Father took the opportunity to say immediately how much James had improved in the last two or three weeks (since I had been seeing him). He was easier to control and was talking and using words (no mention had been made before about his being backward in speech). Mother then suggested they wanted advice, but I got the impression that father was acting as spokesman for a decision that had been made. As he was emphasizing the improvement, and as his wife's interjection seemed to convey anxiety about what he was going to say, because I would feel hurt, I concluded that they did not want to come any more. This inference I put in the form of a statement that it seemed they felt ready to take charge of James again. Mother again interpolated that they wanted advice but father went on to assert: 'As he is now, we should never have come along'. He went on to extol James and said how very clever he was: 'He learns all the tricks'. As might have been expected, he went on to compare himself with his son, evidently enjoying his being so much like himself. My views were not asked, so I did not give them.

It was decided, however, that we would help over finding a nursery school and left it open for the family to return if they thought we could help any more. They did not return but we followed up at the nursery school, where he settled well.

Discussion

There are quite a number of cases that follow this pattern. For it to develop, minimal intervention is required and the family, mainly by making good use of the interviews, succeeds in reorganizing itself in a stable enough pattern. At first sight, James's symptoms were quite alarming but the central one, the restless anxiety, could be managed and with a bit of support in improving her physical health James's mother could, with father's help, become a good enough mother. It was discovered, during a visit to the original nursery school, that it was not the faecal incontinence that had led to James's exclusion but his restless activity; the teacher wanted to avoid offending father by saying James was difficult. James's admission to a better school gave his mother, who was basically a good mother, more time to recover.

This case illustrates how doing as little as possible is important because of the good on-going potential in the family and the child. Interpretation was not required, largely because father was so omnipotent. In another family, knowledge of psychopathology might have been much more useful to them, but in this one only mother and child showed indications of needing help; but it turned out that mother was much too submissive to stand up to her husband and get much of it. To do so would have meant a revolution in her relation to her husband and the couple got along well enough as it was. One reason for so thinking was the rapid recovery of James, which my interviews with him had suggested was possible.

I did not offer the 'advice' for which mother asked because her request seemed to be a face-saver for me when confronted with her husband.

The next case is more complicated and led on to active therapy.

Case Two

FIRST INTERVIEW

Father, mother and two small children came to the clinic because one of them, John, aged two and a half, was said to keep his parents awake at night by head-banging.

According to my usual practice and to test the amount of anxiety about referral to the Clinic, I asked to see John on his own, explaining that I should want to see his parents later (first stress situation).

He was a robust and healthy-looking child who came along without much anxiety; indeed, after taking stock of me, he ran along beside me as if keen to find out what I had for him. We soon reached the playroom, where the social worker was sitting. He settled down almost at once to use the toys and after a short time I left the room, telling him I was going to fetch his parents; this introduced a second stress, which tested his trust of me. He stayed behind with the toys, the social worker being left to cope with any crisis that might arise—none did. (I take this sequence of behaviour to mean that there is an overall good relationship of trust between him and his parents.)

Mother and father are both tall; they sit down and the younger brother, Henry, at once joins John in play. Mother gives a rather good, warm impression and, though she is inexpensively dressed, the effect is agreeable. Father is a 'beat type': long hair, wispy moustache and beard. He wears jeans and a blue corduroy jacket that is rather small for him. Both children run around freely; they make the sand tray the centre of their activities and the play-room soon gets in quite a mess with sand on the floor and the carpet. (The children's activities during this and the next two interviews are of this kind; sometimes they run out of the room and if they are away for long one or other parent gets up to fetch them.) The children incorporate the social worker in bits of play, but not me.

It was mother who started off talking, without being asked, by giving some information; John is two and a half years old, sits up, bangs his head and rocks the cot. 'He likes doing it', she said. It is deliberate and he has started teasing her with it.

At this point the father added that John had lots of energy and, like himself, does not sleep much. When John sits up and bangs he looks terrible, 'he hypnotises himself' and can be heard two storeys down—the family lives in a flat. There is a discrepancy of evidence here, but mother and father do not mind disagreeing, or so it seems. There is, however, a pause after this as if the disagreement might be more important than was shown. I ask how they deal with the symptom. They had thought of most practical means, bolting the cot to the floor and padding it, putting it away from the wall in a different room from where the parents slept. Though neighbours heard the noise and objected, the arrangements made met their objections. It is clear from this that in management John's parents could function well as a unit.

After another short pause, mother starts telling something of John's history. The pregnancy, she says, 'was very heavy'; she had been depressed and irritable, throwing things about. Breast-feeding went badly, the baby screamed, refused the breast and after six weeks he was transferred to a bottle on a flexible routine. I do not say anything and the subject changes to the present. Mother continues: besides the head-banging, John is irritable and throws tempers (rather like herself during the pregnancy, I reflected); if frustrated he can be quite nasty. He makes loud 'ah ah ah' noises and still has screaming attacks. Smacks, mother says, are better than gentler methods. Then father steps in: if you give John a toy, he refuses it in the first place, saying, 'Take it away'; then he accepts it. This is just like him (i.e. father).

From time to time father makes tentative efforts to talk about himself and towards the end of the interview seems on the point of erupting. He says he is a very controlled person and works late at night, also that his own father had a breakdown. This statement of father's struck me, but I said nothing about it since it came right at the end of the interview.

What can be learned from this interview?

Firstly, about the environment:

1. The parents seem tolerant of their children, perhaps over-much so; so it could be that there is too little control at home.
2. They combine well over management (of the symptom at least) and clearly agree to a style of upbringing. When they gave differing but possibly complementary views, there was no clash of opinion and each seemed able to consider the other's view without starting the kind of argument that so often turns distressingly poisonous.
3. Mother and father approach problems in different ways: the mother keeps nearer to fact, father is more imaginative and in a sense more feeling. He seems more than his wife to consider the disorder as serious.
4. Mother seems to express her feeling (probably of guilt?) that the symptoms are connected with the difficult pregnancy and breast-feeding by bringing this in without being asked about it.
5. Father twice identified John with himself, albeit in particular respects, and this might make him tend to side with his son when under criticism. His wish to talk about himself and his hint at a belief that heredity had to be taken into account (his father had a breakdown) needed further elucidation.

Taken as a whole, the environment looks good enough but the early history may suggest that it has not always been so and perhaps is not always so at the present time.

John himself: there is evidence of internal distress, recognized most by father, and this probably stems from the start of his life or early in his relation to his mother.

The self and autism

As soon as the family has settled down, I start off by directing attention to the father; I say that I had been interested in his saying that his father had a breakdown because it might mean that he felt something in himself that was like his father and that might be affecting John. This is repudiated at once; he does not get anxious, he says very emphatically, but he adds that his father took to drink and spent £2,000 on a mistress. He seems shocked and disturbed at my interpretation.

Mother retrieves the situation tactfully by shifting the subject to John, but seems to give indirect confirmation that my interpretation had been meaningful to her. John did 'amazing things' and she describes smearing faeces when he was younger; he also hits his younger brother. She then goes on to say that it is *she* who worries, being anxious about her own irritability, fearing that it would damage the children. Mother having said this in support and protection of her husband, the pattern of the interview repeats the earlier one; mother gives facts but this time father talks more about himself.

The head-banging may follow a smack. Henry (the brother, aged fifteen months) has also started head-banging, in imitation of John. The habit began when John was seven months old (last time it was mentioned, in the first interview, it was six months). Three or four months ago John had a fever; he went into a coma and nobody had any sleep. It was at this time that he ran away from his nursery school.

She talks more about how John could be nasty by taking all the toys away from Henry; I interpret that he had lost his best toy, i.e., his mother: she had been taken away from him by Henry, so perhaps he was feeling the loss of her. Mother replies that she . . . and then she makes a gesture of putting her arm round him. I say I think that sometimes good mothering cannot make up for the loss and I point out that John was only one year old when Henry was born and that this would make it difficult for him (thinking of the disturbed breast-feeding). This leads on to more about John's nastiness to Henry. Suddenly there are rather loud cries; Henry, the younger boy, has got hold of a bit of John's hair and is pulling it; John is helpless and unable to extricate himself. Mother, kindly but firmly, makes Henry stop and comforts John. Because mother had implied that the younger brother was a victim of the elder, I remark that Henry seems able to look after himself in one way at least.

At one point mother goes out of the room, fetching the children who had run out; father then says how anxious he is about mother getting exhausted. He himself works until two or three o'clock in the morning. He is a teacher at an art school and a painter. He had slipped a disc some time back; it was very bad and painful. There are student pressures because of drug-taking. He only needs two to four hours' sleep, however. It is when he goes to bed that John starts head-banging.

Comment

In this interview more information was given about head-banging and other symptoms were added. It began in two situations:

1. After physical punishment by his mother, and
2. When he is left out of a pairing situation, i.e. father and mother together; this was only referred to at the end. There was another pairing between mother and Henry that seemed important but it did not directly stimulate head-banging.

THIRD INTERVIEW

This time I start off by saying that I had been struck by the father's saying that the head-banging started when he went to bed, so I wondered about sleeping arrangements. Suddenly there is a bang. John had got hold of a gun with a rubber-headed missile and had shot his father in the head. Father is startled, protests and takes the gun away. John goes off to play. (Since the children could hear what was being said, I reflected, but did not say, that this attack on father might have been connected with talk last time about father going to bed with mother and John's anger at my asking this time about sleeping arrangements.) It turns out that the parents had recently moved into the room next to the boys. Mother thinks the children have become more restless since the move, but father thinks this is because mother hears more now, i.e. is more alerted to what is going on in the next room. Mother adds here that in bed John cuddles up round Henry, implying that he is able to pair off with and get comfort from his brother and so make up for the loss of mother.

In this interview the mother's anxieties about loss of sleep come more to the fore; to make it all worse John had hallucinatory fears in the dark, saying to his mother 'Look, look, look'. At this juncture mother reveals more of herself: when eleven or twelve years she had had fears of just that sort. There follow more comments by father about illnesses and I then summarize what I had said before and offer treatment for John. Before they reply, however, I take up a rather snide remark that father had made about psychiatrists. I say that I am not sure what he meant by this but perhaps he takes a poor view of them and would not favour further treatment. 'Not at all', he says, and then informs me that as a student he had been sent to one on three occasions by his art teacher because of his open objections to the way his art school was managed. Quite a bit of history follows and finally he goes on to reveal persecutory anxiety and asks me whether I could help him prove that he had not been handling 'pot', because the police are after him and are attempting to plant a false charge that he had handled the stuff. It would be disastrous if they succeeded in their false accusations and he could not find a way of proving that he had not touched any.

Conclusions

1. The head-banging is an indication of internalized conflict but related to external situations; the aggression in it can be reversed (shooting at his father's head). The hallucinatory fears also support the idea that his conflicts are internalized. It was on this basis that I thought treatment was indicated.

2. There are clear signs of the lines of identification on the part of the parents, which needed keeping in mind.

3. The parents can combine well over their child, but mother is the more stable influence in the family, containing, as I would put it, her husband and the children. So long as this continued the family was stable enough but

4. It is under stress from social pressures and might be disrupted.

As to the result: I saw John twice a week and the interviews worked out behaviour like that exhibited in the joint interviews:

anxiety about mother, and sometimes his brother being with the social worker, and anxiety about myself as representing his father. It took about three months for the main symptoms to disappear. The family situation turned out to be complex and difficult to do much about.

Summary

I have rather deliberately given contrasting cases. In this difficult field of practice most families come for help not so much for the solution that we might like to arrive at, but for the alleviation of some distress that has become intolerable. If we can help in alleviating that, something worthwhile has been done, but it is often far below what we should like to achieve.

Perhaps this is the case in all psychiatric practice but it is more so in the case of children because we hope to do something prophylactic, something that will make the child less subject to mental disorder in later life. So it can seem that all cases need treatment of a rather extended kind and how much should not be attempted is forgotten. That at least was what I had to discover before I could limit my aims and understand that dealing with a part of the trouble was more useful than trying to achieve the impossible.

CHAPTER TEN

Child analytical psychotherapy

In chapter eight I reviewed some of the techniques used to treat children psychotherapeutically and contrasted these with analysis. Over the years I have used most of them, but have found them often less satisfactory than applying a modified form of analysis that aims at treating one or more forms of anxiety only, and avoiding affective situations that require regression within the transference. To do this presented a variety of problems to which I can now draw attention. Two of them were related to the nature of the transference and the use of 'deep' interpretations, about which it is particularly important to be clear.

That small children developed a transference was soon sufficiently obvious to me early on in my work with them, but was it advisable to interpret? The danger in so doing was that an undesirable regression would be induced, which could not be managed because cases could not be seen often enough. At that time, in the 1930s, there was a vigorous controversy being worked out among psychoanalysts as to the nature of the transference in childhood. On one hand Klein held that it was not different from the adult's; on the other Anna Freud thought that it could not be the same, because the child's parents were still present in reality. These conflicting views, each dependent upon a different conception of early maturational processes, could not be reconciled. Klein held that an infant developed complex fantasies about his mother that bore little relation to reality and that these soon represented a system that could be transferred to the analyst. The real existence of the parents was therefore relatively unimportant for transference formation.

This view was contested by Anna Freud who, supported by a considerable body of psychoanalysts, thought that the parent-images were derived from the real external parents and were therefore firmly attached to them. Consequently the analyst had to develop an initiatory technique of detaching the imagos from the parents on to himself before a transference could be formed. In this and other respects child analysis, she held, was significantly different from its adult equivalent when the patient was no longer dependent upon nor in the control of his real parents.

From my own position the problem was theoretically not difficult because Jung's concept of archetypes could be used to support the idea that the parent-imagos were primarily as much, if not more, the creation of the child, and so parts of the self, as of the real parents themselves; the development of the personal unconscious would account for Anna Freud's findings. At the time it did not seem to me that there was any necessity for the preparatory exercises because a transference seemed to develop immediately. I now think that such a quandary is due to the failure to differentiate between a transference neurosis and the archetypal transference on which the former may be built and which it may obscure. Therefore my own problem was not so much who was right; it was a correlative one: is it safe to use 'deep' interpretations and particularly archetypal transference-interpretations?

The term 'deep' is a loaded word and has acquired an unnecessary prestige. It refers to something invisible, under the surface, and potentially dangerous; its loading may be due to the intrusion of archaic images associated with the unconscious as symbolized by the sea. The important question that this meaning brings out is whether the unconscious content is accessible to consciousness or no; if it is deep is it safe to bring it to the surface under conditions when 'full analysis' is impossible? Let me illustrate the subject of whether it is deep or near the surface by citing two cases; in the first the affect determining the child's behaviour was accessible, in the second it was not.

Case One

John, aged seven (cf. also p. 116f.), came into my play-room with trepidation. I gave him some toys and suggested he play with them; he did so with a feverish restless activity that made it impossible for him to develop a particular game. The restlessness was characteristic of a child who is anxious and who cannot master his anxiety in play. When I had gone to fetch him from the waiting-room, his mother had said that he should go with the 'doctor', so when alone with him I interpreted as follows: 'I know that doctors often do things to children that the children do not ask to have done to them, so I think you may be imagining me to be a doctor who is going to do something to you that you don't like.' He brightened up at once and agreed with enthusiasm. He asserted that he hated doctors because they operated on him and stuck things into him. As he talked he pointed to his eye, which had a slight squint, meaning that the doctors wanted to operate on him for this.

Later on I learned from him that he had been treated with injections for hay fever, that the injections hurt and that he had concluded from this that doctors did him harm.

The accessibility of the material here depended on overt anxiety and a rather clear clue to its nature was given later by John's mother. The situation made an understandable interpretation possible and this relieved John's anxiety sufficiently for him to give information of some sources for his fears.

Case Two

June, aged eight, took to making rather formal pictures every time she came. She would say scarcely anything about them. After about three months I suggested she should stop making pictures and use the toys: she compliantly went to the doll's house and played a ritual game of putting the furniture in order. In either activity she would finish before time and would stand quietly until the end of the interview. She came regularly and her mother said she loved coming, and indeed this was my own impression.

Case two shows inaccessible conflicts; she gave me nothing on which I could make an interpretation. She herself showed no overt anxiety, only a docile and successful and well-developed passivity. She behaved as if she had no anxiety at all and it was only if one remembered her mother's statement, that she had hated her daughter almost from her birth, that her daughter's passivity and apparent inability to relate to me was understandable. This was probably June's successful adaptation to the situation of 'being hated', but, though I could formulate this idea, the child gave me no clues and no interpretation could be made. When her mother came to the clinic it was probably, in the child's mind, with a view to having something done to the child that she would not like; consequently the important event

vas that nothing happened. In this case the mother had almost
olved her hatred of the girl, and after a few interviews she
ould re-establish her relationship with her daughter, who was
oy then further reassured by her interviews with me.

These two cases illustrate one use of the term 'deep', for in
Case One the anxieties and some sources of them are near, if not
on the surface. In Case Two they are deep down below the
surface and were not relevant.

Interpretations directed to the instinctual libidinal or aggres-
ive roots of the anxieties are indicated only if analysis is to be
undertaken. This use of the term 'deep' is structural and does
not refer to whether the instinctual forms and processes are
deep beneath the surface or no—they may be or they may
not.

In Case One I had interpreted material that was near the
surface, but I had not gone on to make another kind of interpretation that was deep, in the structural sense, i.e. of the
complex being under repression. In short I had not referred to
the castration anxieties, which only came out much later. I
would consider such an interpretation bad technique because it
would not be understandable to the child.

Because of the ambiguity in the use of the term 'deep', which
has done much to put therapists off using appropriate interpretations, it seemed to me desirable to consider in what ways
analytic behaviour is possible or impossible in a child-therapy
set-up. If either of these cases had been coming for analytic
therapy I don't think I should have behaved differently in any
essential respect, except that I should not have suggested that
the girl stop making pictures, and if the need arose I would have
interpreted the defensiveness of her passive resistance.

The object of interpretations is to relieve anxiety and to set the
analytic process going, so if there is available anxiety, as in Case
One, interpretation is relevant; if there is none, as in Case Two,
it is not. In Case One, however, a feature of analysis, the transference and its interpretation, was used in the same way as in
'full' analysis. What then is the difference between analysis and
therapy? The focus is principally on interview frequency. It
may be impossible to see a child every day. In a clinic there are
often special reasons: the psychiatrist or therapist may not
attend every day; if he does, the pressure of cases, most of which
are neither seeking nor requiring analysis, makes it unjustifiable

to spend too much time on one child when so many others are needing help. Next, among those for whom analysis seems relevant, parents may not be ready to make the very considerable sacrifice of bringing a child every day, and even if they are willing to do so, there is the problem of the loss of time at school and consequent interference with a child's education.

All these difficulties combine in varying ways to make less frequent interviewing inevitable and often even desirable. But if the transference is there and can be interpreted, is there any essential problem? So stated there is none, provided the interpretations are used skilfully; but one essential factor is then left out—the working through of resistances. If a child, or an adult, is not seen often enough to work out the effects of some interpretations, the value of them may be lost and the patient will in the interval between sessions built up resistances that are very difficult or impossible to work through. This is particularly so when acting out and dramatization predominate, so that gaining insight becomes impossible.

Case One, Continued

The following case of John, already introduced above, illustrates the problem. He was a lively, somewhat wiry boy with a very quick mind. He was from the start anxious about leaving his mother, but this he could not admit openly, and so he would ask to go to the lavatory from time to time during the interview. He was restless, and it began to look as if more acting out might occur for he seemed only just able to control himself. His play was of a semi-aggressive character, and he became preoccupied with water—turning on taps, playing with various objects, chalks, sticks and a gun, and expressed wishes to drown people (unspecified). As these were punctuated with journeys to the lavatory it seemed likely that he was afraid of his fantasies about his urine.

In this early period he made a remark that was to prove significant. His mother was in the next room and he threw a small wooden brick at the door, saying: 'If your mother dies, you are responsible!'

John then started energetic attacks on the blackboard chalks, which he broke up until no intact ones remained. I interpreted by pointing out his wish to attack his mother with his 'tinkle' urine) and drown her, and said that the breaking up of the chalks meant that he would break off his penis to stop the drowning, lest this should happen to him in punishment for drowning her; this interpretation made him more excited. John told me that I was rude and his play became even more active. It was clear enough that he felt angry with me and wished to retaliate against me, and I told him so (i.e. I interpreted the transference); he then made a violent assault on me, kicking, pinching and scratching, putting all he could into it, so that it became necessary physically to resist and control what he did. But when I did so he became terrified and ran screaming back to his mother. He left the clinic swearing and cursing at 'that doctor'. I understood this to indicate the persecutory nature of his anxiety, which I had aroused; for in his imagination aggression seemed to be associated with magical powers. This incident represents a difference in behaviour between therapy and full analysis. In full analysis there would be more time and I should have waited to make my interpretation until I was more sure of what the behaviour meant. In that case what followed would not have taken place. I refrained thereafter from inter-pretations likely to reach areas of persecutory conflict. Subse-quent interviews were conducted with his mother nearer the scene of action. John resisted any ideas of separating far from her, would rush back to her from time to time and stand beside her, curling his hair with one hand and sucking his thumb with the other. His relation to me was not, however, only hostile, for at times he would come and sit on my knee and wish to be nursed, as if I were his mother.

The following interviews over a period of two months consisted of a gradual weaning process, in which I represented the dangerous object that had to be battled with and who stood between John and his mother. The attacks continued, but though they threatened to become dangerous they never did and I never allowed them to reach their previous intensity. He knew that he could always retreat to his mother, who was on the spot, and gradually we got back to the position where he could tolerate being away from her. His attacks focused first of all on kicking at my legs, next he wanted to attack my cheeks and nose with his hands and nails. A crisis arose one day when he deliberately threw a brick at the window and this was followed by an attack on my eyes, which I resisted. I could now see the

significance of his previous remark in relation to mother. 'I
she dies, it is your fault' may be translated as: 'I am frightened
of my wish to attack her and if she dies I shall have done it
because part of me wants to destroy her as I want to destroy
you; sometimes I feel I have done it and that is awful because I
love both of you'. This conclusion, not interpreted to John, was
supported by his mother, who one day remarked to him when
he came back into her arms: 'I believe you love doctor just like
you love your mum!'

As he became less attached to his mother, he became more
friendly and could respond to any ideas about himself that I
put to him. He became much more interested in his younger
brother and kept some special toy for him to play with while the
brother waited for him during the hour. Before this his relation
to his brother was predominantly hostile, but now he could get
annoyed with him without being cruel. In addition his relation
to his mother improved and his behaviour became more
controlled.

The difficulties inherent in seeing a child like this infrequently
—once a week— must be evident: absence easily equates with
death and so with fears with which the child is left on his own for
too long a period.

Reference to the history supports the severity of this child's
disorder. He was born during the war and his mother was
evacuated for his birth. Consequently the break-up of her home
life made his arrival not so much of a pleasure as she had
anticipated. She was lonely, worried by raids and her maid
left; John was 'starved', lost weight and screamed a great deal.
Supplementary feeding made the situation better and gradually
mother's confidence increased; her milk returned and the child
continued to breast-feed for nine months. There was no trouble
with weaning.

These early disturbances are ones that are likely to have a
more or less serious effect, but the re-establishment of breast-
feeding and the successful weaning is reassuring.

At ten months he was immunized against whooping-cough
and diphtheria and developed an abscess at the site of the
injection, which had to be cut out and plugged. Thus, before he
was one year old, there were two difficulties that must have had
an effect upon him, and to this must be added that, when
cutting his teeth at eighteen months, he developed a large

patch of eczema under his armpit, which lasted for about two months.

When three years old he developed a hydrocele, which was tapped every few weeks until he reached his fifth year. Though his mother tried to explain to him why it was necessary for him to have this done, he was unable to understand and openly thought that the whole procedure was 'her fault'. Thus one way in which he was feeling about his mother came into the open.

When he was five years old an operation was performed for an inguinal hernia. John was terrified and furious. He would not understand why his mother was not allowed to visit him in hospital and was terrified of being in the wards, and specifically feared the anaesthetic. It was when he started to go to the hospital, at three years of age, that he started to get out of hand and attack other children, particularly girls.

One other significant incident was mentioned by his mother. It took place one day when he was out with her. They were nearly run over; following this his mother had a miscarriage and was taken off to hospital in an ambulance. This incident may be considered in the light of his statement: 'If your mother dies, it is your fault'. In infancy and early childhood separation and death are often equated; combining this with John's experiences in hospital, one has no difficulty in understanding how extremely significant this event in his life must have been.

It is clear that the child's improvement resulted mainly from understanding the meaning of his aggression and letting him find out that it was safe to be violent. I had left the transference to develop, but I had not analysed it with him in detail, and I do not think it would have been possible to do so on once-a-week therapy because its structure was so complex.

When his behaviour is compared with the history, as given by his mother, it is at once seen as likely that there were several situations that had not been worked over with him, but most important is the fact of the very early origins of his psychopathology. Much of his aggression referred to castration fears and these had been powerfully reinforced by the incidents with the hydrocele and the operation; yet neither of these reality situations was referred to, nor was his mother's miscarriage. Perhaps with more therapy the links might have been made, but I do not think that the early oral aggressive component could have been reached. So as to reflect these very early situations in a case like this more frequent interviews would have been necessary. One further feature of this case needs comment. The procedure was analytic in principle but relied heavily on the family—especially John's mother—to cope with the affects realized in John. In general, cases treated in this way require a basically healthy family life.

A Note on Aggression

It is very often thought that, since some children seem to improve as the result of the display of aggression, this is desirable in itself. It was not, however, the aggression in itself that was important in John's case, but rather the ideas, fantasies and beliefs connected with it. Some of the aggression was defensive, i.e. that which was directed against dangerous doctors. Other parts of it were dependent upon fears of what his uncontrollable violence would do to the mother he loved; and there were other forms of it that were not worked out, like throwing the brick at the window, which seemed to be related to his feelings about my looking at him. It is these feelings that are important and each one of them needs understanding differently so that their relevance to the past can be understood and compared with the present. In other words, it is the feelings of the child, which give rise to the aggression, that are more important than the aggression itself.

Conclusion

Since the transference can be observed and the main analytic technique for management of it can be used in a therapeutic setting, the way is open to develop therapeutic skills short of the detailed day-to-day treatment known as full analysis. These techniques differ from analysis in their less rigorous and detailed method and, at their best, in recognizing limitations. What they cannot do is of great importance, and in my view this can only be learned by the therapist himself submitting to full analysis and having treated children analytically, seeing them every day; for only thus can a proper perspective be gained.

It is very difficult to demonstrate the difference unless

detailed case studies be embarked upon. Such studies have been published (cf. Klein and MacDougall), and another one will be presented in Part Three, Case One, though Alan was seen only three times a week.

CHAPTER ELEVEN

Notes on the psychotherapy of infantile autism*

Introduction

There are a number of defined ways of treating autism. The children may be removed from home either as an emergency operation or as part of a treatment strategy (cf. Goldfarb, 1961, Bettelheim, 1967). In an institution the environment may be used by adults in varying ways. The one relevant to this discussion aims to let the children regress with the idea that they will, in the course of time, reach the source of their traumata and relive in a more healthy and normal way the earlier situations that caused the disorder.

Bettelheim (1967) has conducted the most thorough long-term project of treating autistic children away from home. By providing consistent and skilful management over years he obtained improvements that appear to be greater than would be expected without the treatment. His study is the most encouraging so far conducted.

The need for special care, so well documented by him, has been supplemented by Winnicott's demonstration that a psychotic child's mother could provide it; he also uncovered splitting processes in a therapeutic consultation with favourable results, which the family could build upon.

To the care and management of regressed states, which in my cases were handled by myself and the child's mother conjointly, may be added two procedures: (a) analytic interpretation of unconscious contents (Isaacs, 1948; Klein, 1946; Rodrigué, 1955; and Tustin, 1972, whose work is strongly influenced by Klein and Bion). Tustin has shown changes taking place related to her interventions. The autistic child studied by her in detail

---

* Previously published in the *British Journal of Medical Psychology* 39. 4. It has been altered in a number of respects.

was first seen by her when he was three years seven months old; throughout the treatment he lived with his parents, who ended the treatment when he was six years five months old. The age at which she conducted the treatment may be important and the fact that in my own case James had entered the latency period may well have contributed to my less favourable result. (*b*) Therapy directed to develop some particular characteristic such as speech (Weiland & Rudnick, 1961) or which aims to draw the child out of 'idiosyncratic activities' by participating in them (Betz, 1947). This technique has disadvantages, but is supported by Mahler (1969), who illustrates it with subtle and ingenious examples.

Care and Analytic Interpretation

The approach I have come to consider most valuable is a mixture of analysis and 'special care'. By 'special care' I shall mean that the therapist aims to meet and respond to the child at a very early level of development and so provide conditions for the self to grow and develop. To do so he required to rely on his own feelings, just as a mother responds empathically to the cues provided by her infant in such a way that the child's own self may be recognized and grow.

Winnicott recently worked on this theme, in a more general context in a paper delivered to the medical section of the British Psychological Society (1965). With John (see below) an incident, comparable to the one he describes as 'bumping up against' the self of the child, occurred. Though usually inarticulate he suddenly burst out one day: 'Fevius [the name by which he called me], you are a b— nuisance', with a force and conviction most unusual in him; he was truly relating to me as a separate object from himself. The child was growing and giving violent evidence of it. The phrase, an expletive that his mother had used about him, was produced when I was interfering with him by acting as he sometimes wanted to, or actually did behave with me or his mother. There was therefore an identification with his mother, which, I infer, his ego actively used for true self-expression.

In the therapy of autism we have to pay especial attention to the relation between social adaptation, symptom loss and growth. That there are ways and means by which an autistic child can be induced to talk, or by which his outbursts can be stopped, by exerting control over them, is not in doubt. Such manoeuvres may be necessary or even desirable steps in management, but they are peripheral to the therapy of autism here defined as growth dependent basically on deintegration of the primary self. It therefore needs bearing in mind that when the child begins to show alarming manifestations this can be a sign of increasing health. Rodrigué (1955), for instance, suggested that the appearance of hallucinations was a clear sign —and in this I agree—that the autism was changing for the better.

In analytic therapy we depend upon verbal communication and so, since the essential characteristic of autism (i.e. the persistent primary self) is that no communication is possible, *analytic treatment of it cannot be undertaken* and therefore care takes precedence over analysis. When we approach the autistic core of a child, his need is to have the condition recognized without intrusive action being taken. This means waiting for deintegration to occur from within the child so that a bit of the self may be discovered, met and reacted to by the therapist. In this area, method or technique are not as important as a capacity in the therapist to tolerate and manage the feeling of being alone, isolated along with a child who gives no indications of his 'presence'.

We have hit upon an issue of much interest. The therapies that depend upon a strategy for bringing the child out of his autistic idiosyncracies cannot be therapies in the true sense, for when they seek to substitute more normal behaviour for the socially abnormal one they violate the need of the self to grow. Yet there are times when the infant needs to be provided by his mother with bits of herself that he can then use for the growth and development of his ego. Thus in the case of the child who called me a 'b— nuisance', his capacity to so react depended on his mother having used these words with affect and conviction. From this it follows that passivity—waiting for a deintegrate to occur, though essential as a base-line for other operations, could be combined with active and affective participation. This point will be taken up later when considering the importance of countertransference affect in therapy.

Social Impact

Gaining access to the self of an autistic child can involve peeling off a number of shells, of which the first is expressed by the members of his environment in a considerable mass of wrong presuppositions about the child. This can have an adverse effect in that it plays on the child's persecutory anxiety, if present, which is thereby increased and he is made by the environment to retreat defensively.

In nearly all cases the nature of the autistic disorder causes anxiety not only to the family but also to the society in which the child is living. A striking instance is that for a long time the diagnosis of infantile psychosis was not made by child psychiatrists because of fear that the words schizophrenia, autistic psychosis, etc., would condemn the child to a bad prognosis. Thinly veiled behind this fear was primitive word-magic but there was, and still is, also something worth being afraid of.

A boy with a rather profuse inner world and marked persecutory delusions improved very much in a hostel and went to school, where he began to learn (cf. p. 175 ff. infra). This happened during World War II, when there was tolerance for bad or difficult behaviour of evacuees. The hostel matron was not told that the child suffered from infantile schizophrenia and she managed the case beautifully. When the hostel closed the child went to another one, the new matron found the child intolerable and a psychiatrist was called in and made the correct diagnosis; the child went to a special unit where he developed an irreversible regression and finally was sent to a mental hospital for adult patients.

This example is fortunately not characteristic, but environmental anxiety expressed in the need to interfere is very noticeable in my cases. In each of them, one or more persons in the child's environment had become destructively excited.

The foregoing remarks have seemed to me necessary because if the mother–child unit is to be treated, the couple will need support and protection at least from time to time, in their joint efforts to lead a bearable existence.

Latterly the diagnosis has been used in a balanced way. It has also been shown that children with what is variously called infantile autism or schizophrenia can recover to become viable members of society. The beautiful example of a therapeutic consultation that initiated the recovery of a schizophrenic child was published by Winnicott (1965). The case depended on making the diagnosis of schizophrenia; it shows, without a shadow of doubt, the advantages that can result and the rapid changes that can take place if the therapist succeeds in uncovering the point of arrest in developing ego structures.

The prognosis is not always socially bad. Indeed, it is common knowledge that children showing marked autistic features can do quite well in ordinary schools. They may have engaged the interest of the teachers, especially when they show unusual abilities of one kind or another or achieve prominence, particularly in academic fields. These children can also provide rewards, sometimes sensational, for those who treat them. Intelligence quotients may rise considerably (cf. p. 254 infra) or parents may provide sustained gratitude. These are the compensations for the very meagre results of our efforts.

Much has been made of the family's environment and of the guilt that mothers of autistic children display, and vigorous attacks have been launched on psychoanalysts who maintain that the condition is caused by failure on the part of the mother to meet her infant's needs. This view, it is maintained, is unwarranted and, by implication, vindictive.

The guilt of mothers is complex and can reach persecutory or even paranoid dimensions. It can be brought out in undesirable ways by unskilful management of it. It is no doubt this that those who object to its being mentioned are talking about, for if, as seems likely, there is some defect in the mother, usually but not always unconscious, it cannot be dealt with by confirming her worst fears: by telling her, for instance, that what she feels is true and that nothing can be done for her child or herself except to recognize the state of affairs.

Management and scientific enquiry are complementary approaches but, whichever is being pursued, it is essential to take the present position into account: a mother needs recognition that she has a child on her hands with which she needs help and who is extremely difficult to live with. This situation is different and more important than how it all began, especially as by the time they bring their children for treatment, many mothers of autistic children can mobilize excellent maternal qualities of care and resourcefulness.

Sources of Material

The observation already used and those to be recorded in what follows are derived:

1. From cases seen for one or a few consultations, often in a crisis. Where a follow-up has been possible, the outcome has been surprisingly good. Sometimes the child's success in adaptation has been largely due to his gifts, the devotion of the mother and a father who is abnormal enough for him to feel that his child's behaviour is within his comprehension.

Cases of children whose own behaviour has necessitated removal to an institution have been rare and occurred when the child's home was emotionally dilapidated. For instance, in one case an attempt at treatment had to cease because the child's mother was unable to tolerate her daughter's behaviour. The rather favourable picture is not representative of infantile autism as a whole but is probably due to the way cases select themselves. Cases hardly ever get referred to me if treatment is manifestly hopeless.

2. From observation of evacuee children in a hostel during World War II. There were two children showing secondary autism; both improved. One entered a grammar school and held his own there. The other started going to school before the hostel closed—the subsequent history was the one detailed above (p. 141). These cases showed clearly the effectiveness of good management.

3. From five cases treated three times a week over 3–5 years —and one followed up by being seen less frequently for $3\frac{1}{2}$ years, making a total of $8\frac{1}{2}$ years. All these cases remained at home though one entered an institution for a short period owing to his mother's going into hospital for an operation. Of these cases:

(a) Two showed secondary autism. They found a way of fitting into society—both changed radically, though in neither had the core of their psychopathology been resolved. Neither presented basic problems in therapy since both were clearly able to use interpretations. The children's behaviour sometimes necessitated physical interventions, such as removing sand trays, and firm action to prevent physical damage to others, so some modification in analytic technique was inevitable. Both children, one

143

a boy, the other a girl, talked freely. The girl's behaviour during treatment corresponded rather closely to the case described by Isaacs (1948) in that very violent and crude 'play' featured prominently in the sessions. The boy's environment was nearest to being 'good enough'. He ranked nearest to the obsessional compulsive end of the scale proposed by Anthony. His treatment is recorded below (cf. Alan).

(*b*) Three showed characteristics of primary autism and it is these that will be discussed in what follows.

The first one was followed up till World War II interrupted communications. He formed personal though limited relationships with the members of his family, talked and fitted into a school for backward children. The second, James (cf. infra), did not become viable away from home though he attended a small group for otherwise ineducable children. By the age of fifteen he had never communicated more than a few words and is still at home attending an occupation centre. The third, John, made considerable progress but his mother terminated treatment, with my passive acquiescence, at adolescence, when he had developed many characteristics of an obsessional neurosis.

The first case (cf. pp. 161 ff. infra) introduced me to the subject and has little scientific value in the present context. I kept notes and some of the pictures that the boy painted in ink but I had very little grasp of what was going on. Looking back, I realize that I was trying to evolve a technique of interpretation and management. The parents and teachers were pleased with what took place but I cannot say whether this was due to a false or true development. In terms of social change the result was better than the second case but I am not at all clear about the state of the child himself.

In the case of James, I deliberately made minimal contact with the child's mother; I wanted to get understanding of the child in the transference alone. There was internal change in that the child became more alive and vivid. The clinic staff noticed it more than I did.

The treatments began at the ages of five, seven and five years respectively. From much of what I shall say about the cases, they will not sound like primary but secondary autism. I contend that this is because analytic treatment was being conducted.

Inasmuch as this is possible at all, the method must have constellated those parts of the self that had developed ego-structures. By using the analytic procedure it became clear to me that, although in these cases of primary autism there had been a basic arrest in development, it was not total. Ego development had occurred, though in a distorted form. This discovery alone justifies the use of the interpretative method. But, further, it is of the clearest value in the management of crises, which occur from time to time. Once a grasp of the areas in which the child's ego operates has been gained, it is far easier to decide whether the affects are derived from the child's mother or arise from the emergence of a deintegrate that, as it were, pushes into the developed areas. When this happens, analysis helps the child to avoid feelings of disorientation.

Interpretative Technique

The technique of using interpretations to elucidate unconscious processes was first combined with observations of children's play by Klein and was applied by her to a schizoid child (1946). Since then the use of interpretations in the way she described has received a wide measure of acceptance and has been sensitively developed by Tustin. It has also come in for critical evaluation (cf. particularly Geleerd, 1963).

Whatever the differences of opinion about the details of how they are employed, the usefulness of interpretations seems beyond question. They are not only the most precise but also the most valuable instrument we have for revealing, penetrating and relating to the structured parts of these children. Apart from the aim of making direct contact with them, studying the effects of interpretation is a valuable research method. That the use of interpretations with autistic children presents difficulties not apparent with others must be granted, and I therefore propose to describe those that I have been able to define with sufficient clarity to communicate them.

In the case of Alan (infra p. 188 ff) interpretations were the main vehicle of communication; with James there were only certain interpretations that communicated and this could be perceived even though he did not talk. In both cases it was the content of the communication itself that was relevant, but there are a number of responses to them which are not so straight-forward. I shall illustrate some of these mainly from a case, John, whom I saw from the age of five years until adolescence, by which time he talked and had developed a clearly defined obsessional neurosis almost exactly duplicating that of his father.

ABSENCE OF RESPONSE

It seems somewhat daring to assert that no overt response to interpretations is a characteristic feature of autism when its core is touched.

It is often hard to detect the effect that a particular interpretation has upon the child. Rodrigué noticed that when he made interpretations of the child's behaviour little or no evident response was discernible. My own experience confirms what he says; there may often be a slight change of expression or an impression in the analyst that something has been heard. But mostly nothing seems to have occurred, though the interviews are producing effects that may be noticed by outsiders, such as that the child for no apparent reason insists on coming to his analysis. The analyst cannot say why this happens, unless it be that he has communicated something felt as valuable by the child. It is therefore difficult ever to say with conviction that the content of an interpretation has had no effect.

There are indeed many pitfalls. Better observation and more accurate assessment of the child's mental life, of which we still know far too little, may be expected to reduce the number of interpretations that appear useless. Also we need to know more about how to use words with a child who may not use them at all. Correct wording can sometimes only be arrived at by trial and error. John, for example, regularly chewed up the legs, tail and head of plastic toys and, as a consequence of interpretations, started to make inhibited attacks in my direction, opening his mouth, raising his arms and jabbing backwards as if struggling to prevent himself fastening his teeth and fingers into my body. At first I referred to '*his* mouth' and '*his* fingers' but there was no understanding on his part and no relief. It was only later when I referred to his struggle to stop '*that* mouth' and '*those* fingers' damaging me that his anxiety diminished.

To establish that failure of interpretations to produce response is characteristic of autism can only be done by producing evidence in favour of the interpretations being correct, and then by showing that these correct interpretations persistently fail to produce any variation of behaviour. This state of affairs was illustrated by John. He showed a number of mannerisms consisting of very rapid and technically proficient manipulation of objects; pencils, pens, glasses, basin plug and chain, soap, etc. The movements of his hands and fingers were highly skilled and even beautiful. The way he picked up the objects was delicate and he assumed an air of distinction as he performed what was to him a highly significant operation to be done with great precision.

The mannerisms were over-determined. Primarily they were masturbation derivatives, based on primal scene fantasies unmistakably acted out in the transference. They were also designed to deal with castration anxieties, and exhibitionistic fantasies entered into them too. But most of all they were magical acts designed to ward off his own violent all-out attacks on his mother, often by projective identification felt as her potential attacks on him. All these components, and others as well, were interpreted as transference manifestations and assigned to their origins either known or reconstructed. Though very occasionally there were slight indications that these interpretations were being used, there was no essential change in the behaviour for five years though other alterations took place. Non-reactiveness of this kind is common and is very impressive: it warrants the postulate that the correct interpretations are experienced by the child as if he and they were one and the same thing. For this reason nothing can happen.

PARTIAL RESOLUTION OF A 'NO RESPONSE'

When this state of affairs is resolving we get changes of the following kind. One day John paid close attention, for the first time, to what I was saying about his mannerisms—in doing so he was distinguishing between two people; when I had completed my interpretations, he remarked: 'Words, talk' in a tolerant but somewhat superior way, making it clear that this was the end of the matter. It is relevant to say here that before this change took place there were others that had been going on in different areas and these may be condensed into one addition to his vocabulary; he had used the word 'no'. Previously 'yes' served his purpose sufficiently. I understand this to mean that he had progressed, in this area, from a state of fusion to one in which boundaries existed (cf. Spitz, 1957).

INTERPRETATIONS IN THE AGGREGATE

Interpretations can be reacted to as a whole and then particular ones take a secondary place. John, for instance, would not stay in the room if I ceased interpreting his activities. If I stopped he would go out. I have not been able to analyse the cause of this with this child but have simply pointed it out to him and reduced repetitive interpretations progressively until some clear change in behaviour appears. An explanation of this could be that the child plays the analyst's game but I do not think John reacted in this way. I believe that my words had become sounds that wrapped him round and he then felt safe. In this sense, their repetitiveness had become important. When they stopped, a radical change had taken place—what was happening? Then the silence became persecutory.

PERSECUTORY INTERPRETATIONS

By contrast, interpretations as a whole may become treated as persecutors or unwelcome intruders. So long as this is understood, the tendency for interpretations to produce persecutory anxiety can be made manageable. I would state, categorically, that a manageable degree of persecution can be positively useful because it gives a clear indication that the interpretations are being related to and can be a clear sign of development and growth. If a child, previously failing to respond, reacts by putting his finger in his ear and rubbing it round as if the words had become objects that he wants to extract, do away with or rub out, anxiety can be reduced by recognition of the state of affairs. John did this and helped me to a much clearer understanding that he was needing me to recognize that I was felt by him to be 'bad'. When I used that word about myself he stopped his activities and looked at me almost incredulously to remark: 'Did you say "bad"?' and nodded his head as if I had at last understood. The door was open to aspects of the child's omnipotence in a way that had not been possible before.

REVERSAL IN USE OF INTERPRETATIONS

This example illustrates another feature of responses. They can depend upon the analyst finding out what the child already knows. The interpretation does not then relieve anxiety by telling the child anything new about himself, but rather gives him information about his therapist's capacity to understand.

CONCLUDING NOTE ON INTERPRETATIONS

Lest it be thought that interpretations are the only way to produce changes in these children, it is sometimes necessary to remind ourselves that verbal methods other than interpretations can be very effective and induce dramatic changes. Geleerd (1949), for instance, showed that a schizophrenic child, in the grip of terrifying hallucinatory fantasies, could be told that they were not true and when a pleasant fantasy was substituted the fears went and the child jumped into her lap. Such examples could be multiplied.

Countertransference

So far interpretations whose effects can be observed have been considered as instruments used by the therapist. They are based on observations and are the result of conclusions arrived at inductively.

Where there is repeated failure to get any response from the child it will be a very tough-minded analyst who does not doubt the validity of what he is doing: are not his interpretations badly timed, too long, too clever, too complicated, or even totally wrong and due to his countertransference illusions (Fordham, 1960)? However much active scrutiny of motives is laudable, there is a limit to it, reached when self-analysis is clearly fruitless. Then it is legitimate to consider whether the feelings and reflexions associated with self-scrutiny are not really something that the child himself is inducing in the therapist; and it becomes relevant to consider whether they might not be a way of compelling attention to the child's own bewilderment, or more likely to that of his mother. If so, this feeling might be reflecting the infant–mother set-up as mothers can sometimes describe it.

This realization leads on to another basis for interpretation that is without doubt important in the therapy of infantile autism. The interpretation is not to be based so much upon evidence observed in the child as upon the analyst's own countertransference.

John played with water and the activity necessitated taking his clothes off. Not wishing to dress him myself (which, however, I did later on) I made an arrangement that I should hand him over to his mother and she would dress him. This she did but it took rather a long time and sometimes involved considerable noise. On one occasion the noise became penetrating enough to be heard all over the clinic and not only caused distress, because it sounded as if the child was being ill-used, but might also have alarmed other parents and children. I, accordingly, went into the room feeling distressed and saw a helpless mother standing on one side of the room holding a vest; there was a naked child running about on the other side emitting peculiar noises whose nature I have never succeeded in putting adequately into words. Something had to be done, so I started from what I felt and said that he was 'putting angry noises into my head that made me want to scream'. He looked at me, stopped the noise and let his mother dress him without further ado.

The value of allowing and relying on countertransference has been noticed by others. Heimann (1950) was the first to do so and Bion (1955) relies on it as a source for interpretation in his analyses of cases of schizophrenia, while Racker (1961) has drawn attention to the importance of how interpretations are formulated and shown that the 'how' can be more important than the interpretation's content. To underline the importance of the phenomena, I have suggested the term 'syntonic countertransference', to be distinguished from an 'illusory countertransference', which ideally should not occur because it leads to interpretations that are relevant not to the child but to the therapist himself. The theory of projective and introjective identification explains the syntonic countertransference and gives it an extra and more dynamic dimension. The point I wish to make here is, however, that affective processes set in motion in the therapist and expressed verbally can be just as and sometimes more effective in promoting changes in the child's behaviour than those that do not contain affect: what the child projects into and so evokes truly inside the therapist, rather than what is known (mentally) or inferred by him, is most usable by the child, particularly when very early infantile oral and anal dynamisms dominate the scene. One difficulty is that the children can evoke such unutterable boredom, rage and despair in the therapist that nothing can be done with it. It was partly to understand this that I continued so long with James. I concluded that much of it was due to the introjection of the child's unexpressed destructive affects and his depression.

With John the problem did not arise but there was another one. There were times when the child was quietly inaccessible, to all appearances. He sat in the chair next to me, with a rug over him and held round his neck, in which he would from time to time bury his face. To me he remained an impersonal object unless I made interpretations known to have been relevant in the past; then he seemed to become a person. It may well be in this area of the analyst's affect that therapy of the autism itself may sometimes begin. When Rodrigué (1955) says of the child to whom he was talking: 'I felt that he was listening to my interpretations. There was a certain alertness on his face that was new to me' (p. 154) he expresses the experience that is most relevant and I think most frequent. As one approaches the autistic core itself, it seems necessary to rely on cues and respond as a mother does to her infant, and to use one's own empathic understanding rather than deliberate inductive inference.

Entering into the Child's Activities

I have already remarked on one way in which I intervened in the management of John. My interpretation resolved a crisis which none the less recurred, so I started to dress the child myself before returning him to his mother. He was quite ready for me to dress him, so long as it was clearly understood that sometimes the clothes became 'bad' and had to be kept away from him till they became acceptable.

In other ways management can become necessary. Excessive amounts of water may get thrown on to the floor or decanted from a bucket and it can become necessary to spend most of the interview mopping it up. These activities, which need handling so as not to become isolating impingements (Winnicott, 1952), are determined by necessity and are not as interesting as those that are deliberately initiated by the child. John insisted on sitting on my knee, robbing my pockets and exploring my mouth, later pushing and pulling me about and initiating chasing or other games with or without the verbal request 'Like to run around and chase me', a phrase that developed from 'run around' and then reached 'Would you like to run around and catch me?'

Sooner or later it will be positively desirable to let these activities happen and to respond to them before stopping them and saying why you do so. They reveal aspects of the child to which access would not otherwise be possible and are true communications. By allowing and following up his physical behaviour it was possible (with John) for me to understand the importance for him of my not having a breast, the fears he had about his having destroyed it magically by stealing it and biting it up and also to grasp his later wish to fill up the hole he had made; he used my breast pocket to fill with objects—mostly plastic toys, which he had previously chewed.

Management of the Mother–Child Identity

Other physical interchanges (including hugging and stroking autistic children) are relevant, but I should feel very uneasy about employing them if I were not clear about it in my own mind and had not communicated my ideas to the child in suitable terms. These activities all belong to care in regressed or undeveloped states. In the case of James I became interested in the fact that he never made any sensual approach to his parents or to me. I therefore tried putting my arms round him and inducing him to sit on my knee. His mother had always managed her physical relation to him competently and he had been the passive partner in it. John was quite the reverse; he would sit on my knee on his own initiative, becoming sensual, using the skin of his face and lips to obtain pleasure. Almost identical behaviour occurred with his mother who managed the situation well, if perhaps too passively. In this behaviour I believe I was representing the child's mother.

It is well recognized that the identifications made by these children are different from those made by more normal children: therefore they are called states of fusion, primary identity or symbiosis (Mahler, 1969). Inasmuch as these states are more than the equivalent of delusions and hallucinations because they are fitted into by the mothers of the children, the mothers may be expected to, and indeed do, play a particularly important part in treatment.

A common feature of the mothers of James and John was

their devotion expressed in bringing them to be treated, though I never held out any hopes of benefit. The second and third both came because they believed that there were other ways of management than sending their children away from home. The reasons given to them by other psychiatrists were not convincing to them and I had only to point this out for both mothers to conclude that they wanted to keep their children at home so long as I would see the child. Whatever delusions the mothers had about the treatment I never gave them any verbal support.

Anthony: (cf. p. 161 ff infra) This mother was by and large a good enough mother during treatment. She had given birth to seven other children and only this one was autistic. He recovered considerably.

James: (cf. p. 257 ff infra) Though his mother had many interviews and showed very good management by organizing her very aggressive and ruthless nature, she never revealed much, if anything, of herself and when she did so she stated the facts, inhibiting affect to a truly remarkable degree. When, for example, she described her child's birth, which occurred at the time her husband, a pilot in the R.A.F. was killed, she never showed a trace of feeling about the situation. When the time came to stop her seeing me, she refused an interview I offered and broke off contact, looking like 'hell'. My own conclusion was that she had adapted aspects of her autism to 'normal' behaviour, becoming a highly competent housewife and business woman.

John: This mother had at first unproductive interviews with the psychiatric social worker and casual ones with me, in which she showed strong paranoid trends. When these had diminished it was suggested she might go into analysis; she agreed but soon developed a delusional transference and left her analyst after some months. She continued to bring her son to me, though any references to her own inner state immediately led to intense persecutory anxiety.

On the other hand, there is no doubt that she has become grateful for what is being done—she says it is the 'only constructive interest that is being taken' and she is consistently reliable about attendances. She knows of my capacity to manage difficult situations with her son apparently better than she can, for instance the incident I have cited over dressing her child, and this had made her feel admiration for and rivalry with me.

This mother had gone to great lengths in the management of her child. She organized her home so that it is at once attractive and suitable for her son. The furniture is strong and the ornaments, unless out of reach of the boy, unbreakable. She and her mother look after him in what is, in effect, a good mental home for one case. Her husband, from whom she is divorced, visits occasionally.

The problem that presented itself was how to manage the mother–child unit and to understand more about its nature. It could not be done by direct analytic approach to the mother, but perhaps something could be done by another method, i.e. by seeing mother and child together.

I therefore decided to instigate some joint interviews with the mother and her son together. One day, when I thought from various slight indications that there was a conflict situation at home, I asked mother and son to come together for an interview. A lot of information was given me by the mother, but her son was furious: he stamped, deployed his mannerisms and went through in a chronological sequence, his mother's most guilt-laden behaviour—to whit, the conflicts that her husband to a greater, she to a lesser, degree had engaged in over their son's constipation—using broken-up phrases that only his mother could understand. It took several interviews with John alone to work through the trauma he had suffered from this interview.

I had seen John's mother on other occasions when I wanted to obtain information of one sort or another; then the child and mother were not in conflict and it had been useful; so it was *how* joint interviews took place that seemed important. One day I noticed that mother looked over-wrought and her son was showing signs of there having been conflict between them. During the interview with the child, he was disturbed and soon wanted to go out of the room. This situation could usually be managed by interpreting the source of his anxiety and, if necessary, following him outside for short periods, but on this occasion, knowing that he had quite strong fantasies (or ideas) of bringing me and his mother together to replace his absent father, I asked whether instead of going out he would like his mother to come in. He said 'Yes' and, though experience in the past had shown that 'yes' was not reliable, I took him at his word because he could now say 'no'.

His mother was glad to come and talk about his behaviour,

how he had become unusually omnipotent and obsessional, noisy, grizzling, violent. She talked about his rapid mood switches, his acute observation, his sexuality—'He always has been awakened from very young', and his 'homosexual' behaviour with his father on his occasional visits upset her son so much; how an awful irritation comes over him and he and she associate it with 'his funny face'; he will come up and say 'Look, mother, I have got that face'. In letting all this be said I assumed that I knew the boy's mental operations well enough to keep in touch with what he felt, so I could follow, and make interpretations to relieve anxiety as occasion arose. This joint interview was profitable and not traumatic to the child.

The idea being tested here is to look for cues from the child which will indicate the times that he can tolerate or want me to make contact with his mother. As we shall now see, it may be that this can do more than act out the boy's wishes.

Some interviews later, the boy was sitting in the chair beside his mother in the waiting-room, with his coat held up before his eyes. As I came forward to take him for his session he did not move; so I sat down and gave his mother an opening—no other parents or children were present. She told me with even more vigour than before how frightful he had been: for three hours he rampaged about the house stamping backwards and forwards, commanding things to be done for him, reducing her 'to pulp'. (I knew that when he did this in the transference it was a defence against the—to him—terrifying attack he was feeling impelled to make with mouth and hands.) Further she detailed how he had been terrible on the bus, talking nonsense in a loud voice and, when he got off the bus, he rushed away from her, so she had kept him back from 'school' (he attends an occupation centre) till he had calmed down.

The substance of interpretations I gave was as follows: the nonsense talk was to counteract the noise and rhythm of the bus and the talk of the horrid people on it. When they got off the bus she became a bad mother, which the horrid people on the bus represented before. John, meanwhile, dropped the coat from his face; a cardboard tube was protruding between his legs like a large penis.

His mother went on talking about his commands. He commanded a drink, the kettle must be put on and in the right position, it must boil at once or he got angry with it: various actions, previously to be done twice, must now be done several times till he is satisfied—he *can* be satisfied, I am assured.

She recorded how she tried to accommodate herself to John's omnipotence and up to a point succeeded, but sometimes her limit was reached and then she would become furious and shout, but he only enjoyed it and laughed (six months ago she had reported that he was terrified of her anger). Here she went on to talk about her own position, and used an automatic-sounding phrase, 'I must look after myself'. Her son's future was harrassing her and she seemed to compel herself to introduce harsh realities: no good school will take him, all the places he could go to are so awful she cannot send him away. What she can give him is all he will get and then there is the mental hospital to which he could go *as an adult*, and she hastened to say that her son could not understand what this was like; I interpolated that I thought he did know in his own way. (Something had to be said by me here to disidentify me, in the boy's eyes, from his mother's obtuseness.) I remarked that she only tormented herself with realities because she loved her son so much that she would not part with him. She then told how her mother took over from time to time and they looked after the boy in shifts; her mother 'is not heartless as she used to be.'

During this talk the boy brightened up. He passed flatus—his mother protested mildly—then he picked up the cardboard tube and walked off manipulating it; 'Shall we go?' he said to me, and mother then revealed more about herself. She had had a shock: her boy-friend—whom she was going to marry—had died, and she said this in such a way as to imply that her son was being felt to express her own desperation. I followed John into the play-room, where he said, 'Will you run around?' and a recurrent game ensues. When I became worn out and sat down he pushed and pulled me but I did not move and he started his mannerisms, walking about.

Next day the mother says that the crisis, which had been continuing for about ten days, is over. In my interviews with him, John's anxiety was much reduced.

The idea of developing a technique of seeing mother and son together, but following clues given by the child with a view to handling the contents of their conflicts, is for me a new departure. My impression is that it can only be of value when a conflict is emerging and on the point of being resolved. It is not therefore likely to prove useful in making inroads on the essential core of autism, a view that confirms the idea that true deintegration can only be met in a two-person situation.

Once a grasp has been gained through interpretative work of the child's psychodynamic processes, the autistic core of these children remains basically intact. In no case that I have seen or treated has it resolved, though it has modified itself. The conclusion seems inevitable that the need of autism cannot be met by any means yet discovered. This is what makes these children basically so intolerable to their mothers, from whom they yet can evoke such extraordinary devotion. That this devotion needs delusions such as those expressed in 'I don't think there is anything wrong with him' is not surprising. The devotion, as far as my limited observations go, contains a delusion with whose help, if I may so put it, therapy can occur and I infer that this is because it supports the state of very close identity between mother and child.

To treat a delusion as a basis on which therapy can be undertaken runs contrary to usual conceptions. That techniques and method need to be used by the therapist to participate in a delusion is indeed almost shocking and so it must be added that he need not collude in the delusion if he knows what he is doing.

Conclusion

It is sometimes said that therapy is of no use in infantile autism. It all depends on what is meant by therapy. If by it is meant the facilitation of mental growth then therapy occurs. Indeed the three autistic children who have been discussed here all grew but two of them not enough to satisfy the environment. It is my impression that in the autistic children under review more happened than with other children in therapy, and that it is because not enough happens that therapy is often judged useless.

PART THREE

INTRODUCTION

In the previous section of this book I have been at pains to outline the techniques that I employ in treating children, and in this section I shall present case studies in infantile autism. Only one of these, Alan, was analysed in the stricter sense of the term, but it will be apparent from my earlier statements that all of them, except those who were observed in a hospital for maladjusted children, were approached in a sufficiently similar way to make the data obtained comparable.

Case studies in autism

The following studies of autism (pp. 161–288) were presented in a seminar at the C. G. Jung Institute in 1957. They were designed to show Jungians that there could be a psychopathology of childhood that was not much influenced by the parents. In the first case, little therapy was done with Anthony's mother and certainly none of the kind that Jung's thesis would require. The cases that follow were living in a special hostel for children evacuated, mostly from London but from other cities as well, during World War II. They were separated from their parents, who continued to live in the towns.

The demonstration of child psychopathology is no longer needed, since its existence is now recognized, but these seminars contain so much matter that still bears reflecting upon that it seems worth publishing them. In any case, they represent my jumping-off ground for the more detailed studies I have made of Alan and James, recorded in this volume. None of the cases described in this chapter were being analysed, but Anthony was seen for psychotherapy regularly once a week over about two years.

The text has been somewhat, but not essentially, revised.

Case One—Anthony

Anthony was seven years old when I first saw him. He had been brought by his mother because of almost complete failure at school. The schoolmistress reported that when he came back from an absence, following nasal diphtheria, 'he wailed and cried in a peculiar manner'. He was a year at school before he could say his own name, and after two years he could not produce more than two words at a time. He seemed incapable of learning and, though he would sometimes play with other children, he did not seem to get into contact with them. The impression he gave was of a solitary child who, in the teacher's words 'never gives any trouble but is quite passive', meaning that he would comply with anything that was required of him. His school attainments were negligible, but he liked singing.

There was only one activity that he could not bear and that was teasing, which caused him to cry and scream.

This description illustrates some of the characteristic features of the disorder. The isolation is not just the inward turning of an introverted child; it is virtually a complete absence of relationship to others, so much so that it has been compared to foetal behaviour. Lauretta Bender emphasized the isolation and combines it with the compliance that she calls 'primitive plasticity'. She draws on the studies of intrauterine behaviour collected by Gesell and goes so far as to say, 'Gesell's description of the foetal infant's behaviour . . . represents a description of a schizophrenic child's behaviour through infancy and childhood'. It may therefore be of interest to speculate here that Anthony's foetal life might have been disturbed. He was not a wanted child; his mother became pregnant for the seventh time when his father lost his good position as manager of a department store during the depression in 1926. The whole family was poverty-stricken and the mother was undernourished: she hoped the child would die. But after the birth, which was 'normal', her hatred for the child sank into the background and she felt love for him; she breast-fed and weaned him without difficulty. She noted, however, that he seemed 'more peevish' than her other children.

I may remark here that this mother's anxiety about her effect on her child when in utero must be set in relation to another interesting and more easily accessible idea that children like Anthony do not react to the outside world because it does not exist for them; it is negatively hallucinated. This is a more dynamic idea, though the two concepts are not contradictory.

There can be little doubt that Anthony's mother had considerable guilt over her death wishes directed towards the child inside her, for she never mentioned them to anybody, not even her own mother, to whom she was closely related and usually 'told everything'. Because of her guilt she may well have over-compensated and showered an excess of love on this child, which possibly bound him to her more than the others.

There is a special relation that autistic children develop to their mothers, so much is certain; but I think that not enough is yet known to assess whether it is the consequence of the child's disorder or not. When I demonstrated this case to a group of Jungian analysts in London, one of them remarked what horrors there must have been in the mother's unconscious. Of this there was insufficient evidence; indeed the death wishes and the guilt were all conscious and comprehensible. It is not likely that they alone produced Anthony's psychopathology.

Anthony liked music. This is not unique; another schizophrenic child in my care sings. He knows a lot of songs that he will substitute for speech and he also makes up a number of his own songs. A third, Richard, was fascinated by words and would make up poetry, some of it quite good.

Anthony showed positive qualities. Autistic children, in spite of their isolation, are often remarkably attractive; they may have charm and even beauty; they often have special gifts, artistic or constructive, and it is probably because of these that they tend to attract people to them, so that mothers, teachers, or analysts often seem willing to give almost unlimited time and care to them. Rodrigué remarks on this and connects it with the good object located within the child.

Anthony had no other particular gifts except that he drew goodwill towards him. He was loved by all his family, particularly by an elder brother, aged eleven, and his little sister, two years younger. His father, a hot-tempered Irishman with all the superstitions that go with this type, never resented his lack of performance. He expressed his feeling for the child by saying that he must be lucky, for he was born at seven o'clock in the evening on the seventh day of 1927 and was the seventh child of a seventh child. Only one other significant historical fact was communicated by his mother: when he was two years old, his younger sister was born; she then noticed a difficulty in his 'getting words out'.

Before going on to consider parts of the treatment I undertook, I want to make a speculative interpretation. The child had a kind of wall round him through which it was almost impossible for strangers to penetrate. The only clear response was to teasing, a form of persecution. It may well be that this points to an essential feature of withdrawn children: for some of them most of the outer world is filled with persecuting 'devils' against which they erect a defensive wall that surrounds them; at the same time it protects their ideally good inner world against the bad outer one of which they are unconscious—it having become unconscious through negative hallucination.

But this does not cover the whole of Anthony's behaviour: he had apparently succeeded in emerging from his shell far enough to play with other children at school and in having something of a relation to his elder brother and younger sister. In saying that he had emerged, it could also be said that he made these other children part of himself. I do not know which is true—it might have been either or both.

My Experience of Anthony

I shall now record some of my experiences of Anthony. At the time I tried to understand what was going on, but it is only in retrospect that I understand as much as I have put down here.

Anthony said nothing consecutive for eight months—he was seen once a week—but then he began to talk and his mother reported that his speech became almost normal at home, though he had not yet spoken to me. I observed his activities and tried to participate in them, but no action on my part led to any significant response that I could observe. I tried to say what I thought he was feeling, mostly in relation to his mother, since it seemed that he had hostile feelings to her, but he did not appear to hear it. After many months he protested that I was 'not to say that about his mother' and those were almost the only words he spoke to me.

Soon he became interested in my pipe and this led to making fires. He would collect pieces of paper, often quite large ones, and burn them, thus presenting a difficulty in management. If prevented in potentially dangerous acts he would stop altogether. At this time, his mother said she could not prevent him from making fires until she good-naturedly threatened to burn him if he went on.

I eventually managed this problem by providing a large tin and then his play began to change: he rolled up pieces of paper and tried to smoke them like a cigarette and gradually his aim became clear: he wanted to smoke, as I did, and one day he seized my pipe and tried to fill it with paper so as to make the kind of fire that I made.

Sadistic impulses emerged at this time. He would light a stick and try to make holes in the wall or in other pieces of wood with it. In this he was, I conceived, obliquely expressing his cruel impulses towards me, wanting to bore a hole into my body and burn up what was inside. At this time his mother observed that he would adopt a bullying attitude towards her—'as some men do', she said; and, further, he had started teasing and torment-ing other members of his family and other children as well. Some months later, when I stopped him smearing some paint about, he attacked my penis. When I prevented him he tried to pull my hair, then my nose, and this led to a fight, which ended in almost a friendly manner.

Reports from home over this period were positive: he was beginning to learn, starting to write and to learn his arithmetical tables. His mother also said his relation to his father had become much better; he went out into the garden with him and helped in digging, showing great interest in plants, wanting to know how they grew and what his father did with seeds.

Further, he developed concern over animals that were hurt. He found a little bird that was hurt and abandoned by its mother; on this he lavished infinite care, fed it, and looked after it in a box. On another occasion, he was concerned about a bird that had been killed by a cat, saying, 'She need not have killed it, she was not hungry'. Both these acts were in striking contrast with his previous lack of concern either for others or himself. With me a new development took place: making fire became associated with wanting to urinate; he would hold his penis and rush to the lavatory when making a fire. This would be followed by his washing himself for a longish time.

The Pictures

It is not easy, by purely verbal description, to give an adequate account of how this child behaved.

The pictures started as follows: he had dabbed some paint on the wall and I then put up a large piece of paper, which stimulated him to picture-making. Some of the painting was done with great care; for instance, the portholes of the ship he drew had to be just right—if he started spacing them wrongly he would correct what he had done; but on the whole the pictures were made rapidly and in a state of excitement.

The first picture had three figures in it, the top left hand one showing circular movements in the body.

The second image showed whirling movement in the lower of two compartments, the top one of which was empty. Below was an almost aesthetic figure resembling a hermaphrodite, without arms, though it looked as if there were two embryonic ones on the front.

There was a two-month gap between the first picture and the next—a ship: the first of a series. The second was different from the first in being horrific. A pole standing up may have been associated with his preoccupation with long objects: he would be found carrying a long pole about with him in the street and on one occasion he rushed out of his home, and was brought back by his sister, carrying a board he had found that was much larger than himself.

Red portholes perhaps associated with the fascination traffic lights had for him, the red representing danger. He would stand for long periods looking at them, but he hated to be seen doing it. He was observed, by a friend of the family, looking at the traffic lights when they were against the traffic, i.e. when they were red. He 'shot' into a drapers' shop and hid, peeping round the corner of the door as the tram went by with the family friend in it. This was the first time anything like fear had been described, though during this period he began to look terrified for no apparent reason; it was as if he had imagined or hallucinated a terrifying figure.

The blackness of his ship was the horrific part of it, but perhaps the sense of a fire inside it increased this feeling. I was impressed by the fact that after painting this picture he ran a fever and was in bed for two days, so it would seem that the ship did in some sense represent his body-self.

On the top of the ship was something like a chimney, which made it look like a kind of evil breast (some of the later pictures emphasized the mouth). That the black colour was connected with fear and violence may be confirmed by his covering a whole sheet of paper with black, then tearing it up into small pieces and throwing the bits away. The black may well have been connected with what we have referred to as a negative hallucination. Is it going too far to assume that this terrified him and made him put on the electric light? It may have seemed as if everything was going black.

There was a ruthlessness about his behaviour at this time: he picked up a female doll and burnt the dress. Following this, he destroyed another set of pictures and threw the female doll out of the window. In the same interview he attacked a baby doll and threw it too out of the window. But when all these activities were completed, he would do something towards making good the damage; for instance, he went and fetched both the dolls back again.

There was water in the picture and this also concerned him at the same time. He used to go to the lavatory and it was not only to urinate; he turned on the tap and watched the water come out, letting it fill the basin, after plugging up the drain pipe with paper. When the basin was full he swished the water out on to the floor. Then again he started making good by taking a brush and cleaning up. Later on he started putting water into pots, pouring it from one to the other, or drinking out of them.

How are we to understand all this? Are we to assume that the picture represented just the inner condition? This is too simple, for there was evidence of a great deal of *participation mystique* in all that was going on: the boundary between inner and outer seemed absent or very hazy. We assume that previously there had been a barrier round him—a commonly held view of autism—and that this was now breaking down. Part of his fear might have been that the idealized inner objects so far safeguarded by the barrier were now threatened; and so he felt both inside himself and around him all sorts of bad and terrifying objects.

I refer to them particularly as objects because it is sometimes held that autistic children live in an inner world; while this may be true, it is not easy to decide whether this should be applied to mean an inner world of imagination or no. Everything that has been described about this child, up to the time when he started to paint pictures, had been in terms of objects: in terms of his isolation from people or his relation to animals, toys, fire, water, my pipe, etc. Only as he starts to show signs of fear and paints pictures can we begin to see something that we recognize as primitive imagination; when his fear became terror, imagination had probably reached hallucinatory intensity.

His behaviour is something like that described by Jung as introverted sensation. This is a type that needs the external object to lead him to the inner world of imagination, but here the imagination does not separate from the object, which is thus completely identical with the image. In the same way, the inner world seems to be extremely concrete and elementary, as if the postulated idealized good inner object were *only* physical. This would make it understandable that he got a fever in time of crisis; there is little separation here between a psychic crisis and a physical one. In confirmation of this, a regression took place; later he became ill and it was thought to be appendicitis. When I went to see him in hospital he was lying more passive, inert and compliant than he had ever been. He was running a fever with only a mild infection, if any at all. In this extreme regression he showed a characteristic of other autistic children: they react according to what we might expect to be their inner condition.

Taking the red inside the ship as his first attempt at an image of danger inside him, we can see how it leads to very concrete forms of attempt at release—masturbation, urination and destructive impulses. All these are primitive means of release without imagination. The pictures and quasi-hallucinatory fears may therefore be thought of as a development like other positive forms of behaviour already noted.

I should like to refer here to the interesting comparisons that can be made with passages in Jung's masterly chapter, 'The transformation of libido', in *Symbols of transformation*, where he discusses fire symbolism at length. He links it up with instinctive behaviour on the one hand and spiritual and cultural vitality on the other. In this chapter he brings in the concept of pre-sexual disposition, masturbation, boring holes, speech, fire-making, etc., and relates them to rhythmic activities as a whole. He says: 'It is probably no accident that the two most important discoveries which distinguish man from all other living beings, namely speech and the use of fire, should have a common psychic background.'

To continue with the pictures, I have already referred to the black one that was destroyed. The next ship was very much the same but less black and the portholes were pink; there was a flag in the place of the chimney and another one at the left-hand end; there was more water and in it were some red objects that he called fishes; behind were the four letters A, B, C and D in pink.

The fourth picture was rather different. There were two boats; the one above was a boat with a lattice-like side; over the top was a face with arms coming out of the head. The mouth had three teeth. Below was a steamer, again with four portholes; the superstructure was composed of eleven decks and two funnels. There was no red or pink, but in the left porthole was a little figure, now free to get out—one might consider that the free face above represents this possibility achieved. A process of liberation and differentiation can be inferred from all this. It may be significant that a steamer suggests a fire under control; the decks suggest stairs, and it is of interest that later on he initiated a series of games centred on climbing up and down a ladder going up on to the roof, and later on there was a game of rushing up and down stairs with another boy in the clinic with whom he made friends.

The fifth picture was largely destroyed, but some of the pieces remained. This time it was easy to infer what made him destroy it. In the upper right hand corner was a horrific face; upper left was a single stroke and between them, extending the length of the paper, were ink-smears; below was the little figure seen earlier in the ship. In one of the areas was another face. It had a black outline and a mouth with teeth in it; he painted the face red and then returned to the mouth to make the teeth blacker and thicker, but he had too much ink on the brush and it ran, making a streak down the paper, spoiling his picture. Immediately he tore the paper off the wall; he tore it in pieces, doing away particularly with the red face.

Two things in this picture pointed to the cause of his anger: there was no objection to the black line or the smeared ink, they were both intended, so it is not hard to see how much this child was concerned with controlling what he did in painting; any spontaneous interference with his effort resulted in violence. It did not essentially matter whether it originated from others or from within himself. His passive compliance, the opposite of this violence, can thus be classed together, for compliance as well as violence contributes nothing to what is being done.

The multiplication of images continued in the last picture. The ship had become small, the portholes reduced to three and its flag, a Union Jack surrounded on three sides by a squiggle, had become larger. Below the ship was a tree. On the left was a peculiar figure something like a kite—it started with a cross and this had a special meaning for him. The Christmas before this picture was painted, four months before, he had come home with a wooden cross. It was not known where he got it from; he was very much interested in it and asked what it was for. He was specially keen to know about Jesus and his crucifixion; the nails, which made holes in the hands and feet, were particularly impressive to him. He kept this cross and hung it over his bed.

These pictures, together with the play and behaviour I have described, give us some insight into the structures and the dynamics of the kind of autism that Anthony exhibited.

I started introducing the idea that there is a good internal object, defended completely against a persecuting world. This was in the main denied, in a very radical way which may be compared with negative hallucination. It may have been—in part at least—his interviews with me that changed the pattern of his behaviour so considerably and made him active and destructive. I do not know whether it was through creating a situation in which there was a minimum of interference or whether it was some of the things I said.

It seems quite clear that he started relating to the objects in my room, and I think to me, but as an object rather than a person. He found he could do things without dire consequences, and there was no objective reason why he should have become terrified. Therefore the feared object must have been a reflection of a bit of himself. It is possible to understand the fear if it is assumed that his original condition was pathologically stable: the good object had become almost completely protected, shut off and enclosed so that it was not known about even by him; it was isolated from all his own bad affects—mainly impulses, for at first he seemed to have no imagination as we know it.

No good object had so far appeared in his interviews, but they had appeared at home in the little bird that he cared for, and which he mothered as if it were himself. There are some grounds for the belief that this good object was also connected with his mother, for when I had told him on several occasions and in different ways that I thought he sometimes felt like attacking his mother, he suddenly said; 'I want it not to be said about my mother'. Here the good object seemed clearly related to her because he wanted nothing against her, but in each case the good object was outside him.

Reviewing the history in this light, the fact that the mother felt love for Anthony after his birth, and that the child's breast-feeding went well, becomes especially meaningful because it was '*good*'. So the good object may have been the breast. The only possible good object in his clinic activities was the water, which may be understood as representing his bountiful mother-breast. All his behaviour, and especially the lack of symbolism, points to a very early arrest in his development. Furthermore, what is often described as a good breast-feeding is not necessarily satisfactory, because it often lacks aggressive relatedness; there is no attack on the breast and no bite, the child lies passive in its mother's arms and simply sucks. There is much more in breast-feeding than that.

That his anxiety and aggressive defences were inhibited (except for screaming) is clear, and that his fears were quasi-hallucinated has been suggested; but apart from the breast that had to be kept good and then idealized and preserved, can we see anything else in his behaviour to support it? When he was emphasizing teeth he tore up his picture because something had happened outside his control. Furthermore, in his faces the mouth was particularly emphasized—it had a schematic appearance and was, as it were, mechanized; at the same time, the mouth was open. This suggested inhibited oral sadism and supported the theory of his preventing at all costs the sadistic attack on his mother which he had been acting out in a modified way by adopting his father's bullying style.

If this analysis is the correct one, we must assume that the appearance of his anxiety, his destructiveness and his hallucinations represent a split in his psyche; the good object has been preserved, locked away, as it were, while he releases the dangerous fires that might threaten it. These experiences are all projected into objects, even the pictures must be classed as projections, but in doing this he has begun to form images that are more plastic and of which more appear. In the paintings, for instance, he started from one object and ended with three on one piece of paper.

One other significant feature of his behaviour may be mentioned: his attack on and rejection of the dolls—it was at the birth of his sister that the symptoms were first noticed—may have been fired off by jealous anger of the sort he dramatized in his play and have led him to the deeper regression that seemed to be at the centre of his autism.

But even if all these changes have occurred, if he has become able to imagine, and so form images of an essentially psychic or mental nature, and even if his talking has developed, even if he can now learn, can write, do simple arithmetic and make relationships with other children, the essential split in his personality still remains. This was shown when he was engaged in any concentrated activity of his own. When digging in a sandpit, for instance, he could not allow anybody else to join in; violent hostility would be evoked.

Though his mother reported a relapse, the advances he had made continued. He was a backward child, but no reliable intelligence quotient was obtained. He was moved to a special school for retarded children and settled down there well enough. This was when he was twelve years old; then I lost sight of him when the war started in 1939 and have not heard of him since.

The study of autistic children is interesting in many ways. It is not just their psychopathology that I want to investigate, with a view to eliminating it or making them well, though this comes into it. I have my own quota of autism and this work helps me to understand that; but I have ideas about early ego-development and have related this to the functions of the self as the originator of the ego. I have assumed that the self deintegrates to make the early archetypal forms. How far this view will prove useful I do not know; it could be investigated by studying babies, as Piaget has done, or it could be useful in understanding autistic children because they are so regressed.

Our research into the workings of Anthony's psyche has led us to assume that he was related to what we can now call numinous objects and that all images were contained in them, so that there was none of the ability to abstract from the object found in introverted sensation. Then it seemed there was something that I termed hallucination—if it is not that in the psychiatric sense, it is a very intense image that has the same quality as the objects. Only later did fantasy-images appear, which had a striking analogy to known archetypal forms.

This case gives us the opportunity to discuss what an object is to an infant and, since these are the substances through which archetypes are likely to express themselves first, we cannot avoid a diversion into theory. In the first place, infants know little of objects as we know them. We can get some idea of infants' objects that can be obtained from the study of instinct in animals. Researches into instinct have been collected together in a book by Tinbergen, and it is from these that what I have to say about instinct is taken.

It is known that instinctual behaviour is a release-manifestation. The pattern of behaviour termed instinct is laid down within the organism before birth and is released by a special precise mechanism—the innate release-mechanism. For instance, when a baby gull stands below its mother's beak to receive its first feed, it is not the sight of the mother gull that excites this activity, nor the mother's beak, but the red colour in a circular mark on the beak—it is not the shape of the red mark, only the red colour. This red colour is called the sign-stimulus.

When, therefore, a baby starts to feed at the breast it is likely that there is a sign-stimulus that starts him feeding. It would not be a breast, or a nipple as such. I emphasize this because it would seem that the sort of consciousness that an infant has is most unlike anything we know of, but it is not necessarily *hazy* but remarkably precise. It does not last long but only serves to release sucking behaviour in the infant. This resultant behaviour is mostly innate, though there are individual variations, because a baby is a person as well as an instinctual mechanism. Once breast-behaviour starts, all sorts of conscious forms begin to develop and we can get an idea of what these are like from Piaget's work.

If the infant's initial relation to the breast is made through a sign-stimulus, he soon gets a sense that his mouth is a thing into which objects can be put; he has indeed probably realized this in utero, for children suck their fingers there through the operation of a reflex action. The mouth now becomes the centre of what Piaget calls an oral schema.

These schemata—there are others besides the oral one—interested me because they are so total that there may develop a kind of mouth-world; every 'object' is put into the mouth if possible, or if impossible an attempt is made to do so. The world, inasmuch as it can be called a world, is built up round the mouth, and this must be closely related to the feeding instinct, even though the activities are different from feeding. There are, as I said, other schemata, visual, auditory and prehensile schemata. To my idea, the quality of wholeness of these schemata is an early expression of the self, though in a deintegrated form.

At first the objects have no permanence; when in the mouth they exist, when outside they cease to exist. Only gradually does the object get permanence and only gradually does a concept of space and time develop through the interaction of the schemata, each of which develops by processes of assimilation and accommodation. By permanence is meant that the object is still believed to exist when outside the sphere of immediate sense perception.

The development of consciousness at this very early stage seems to be based much more on experiment and deduction than on fantasy, so that, to put it very crudely, the infant is much more of a scientist than of an artist.

An important event in development is the discovery of what is 'me' and 'not-me', because then there can be a me into which objects can be taken and organized in various ways, and there is a not-me from which objects can be taken and into which they can be put—the primitive form of this is presumably eating and excreting.

The place of imagination in all this is not clear; it looks as if very primitive fantasy, hallucinatory in character, occurs in the first few weeks of life, and that a very important part of it centres on the impermanence of the objects, which are represented as magical through their spontaneous activity, probably hallucinated or something of that kind. This produces a number of terrifying or other affects, which are described as good and bad for want of better terms. These two classes of objects and their magical activity form centres of conflict, anxiety and satisfaction. Attempts are made to preserve the good objects and to master or do away with the bad ones. One such attempt is to put the good ones inside and keep the bad ones projected, as we have suggested happened in Anthony's case; only we should have to assume also that he regressed to the condition where there was no outer world, in order to do away with the bad objects. An important point is that, though the earlier stages in development are in a sense superseded, they also tend to become represented in the later forms of development; partial or complete regressions can occur.

Before turning to more case material, I want to say something about the nature and use of this theoretical reconstruction. It is not 'true', its only value is to orientate us. It is for this that we make theoretical models; they are models to which we refer and which bring a measure of order into the material we examine. Everybody who interprets material has a model in his mind, and I have outlined my model not because it is to be believed in and not because it is complete, but because it is necessary to give a statement about the thinking behind what I say.

LIVING IN A MAD WORLD

Two Cases of Schizophrenic Children observed in a Hostel during World War II

The case material I now want to present was provided by two boys: one, Richard, was aged nine, the other, Charles, was six when the observations were made. They have this in common: they were both complex personalities who developed together imaginary worlds in which they each lived; but the outcome was radically different in that the elder won a scholarship and did well, while the younger ended up in a mental hospital. The description of each will of necessity be incomplete; indeed it will be confined to the investigation of their worlds and of other children's attitudes towards them. I have decided to include these two cases in order to illustrate and give the flavour of the kind of imaginary reality that some autistic children create for themselves.

Both these children were first seen by me in a hostel for abnormal children. The younger one developed his world first; it was called Lighton and he lived almost completely within it, so that if the hostel staff wanted to control him they had to learn the language of this place. The language was called 'Litish'. At times nothing could be done with him without this knowledge, though he could at other times speak normally. When he came into a hostel he fascinated the other children and they all started to make up inner worlds of their own. But only these two did more than just play with this world-making activity; one was Richard, the other was Charles, who had started it.

Richard, aged nine, was at first apparently a very aggressive and terrified boy, who caused a great deal of difficulty at meal times. Many of the foods placed before him were violently rejected and some were thrown about the room or at other children. This was because, as I discovered later, he had equated the food with sewage and faeces, both of which were felt to be dangerous, i.e. bad for various reasons—for instance, because of their colour, smell or shape.

One day he was put to bed because of his behaviour and I went to see him; he announced that he was a ghost and that therefore I could do nothing to him. So I started a game in which I said that I was a more dangerous ghost than he was because I was mad. I continued by saying I was going to eat him up, then put the light out and I pretended to look for a soft piece of flesh to start eating. He remained unperturbed, however, and talked ghost language to himself. This game was remembered for a long time with pleasure, and whenever I visited the hostel he would come up and say: 'You are still a ghost, aren't you?'

When the imaginary worlds started Richard became particularly interested. He had many excretory fantasies and used rude words as power words, though sometimes urine and faeces were referred to as lemonade and chocolate. Charles also liked this and in secret they could be seen finding bad smells wherever possible and making up long lists of things, written on lavatory paper. These lists were not to be seen by grown-ups and so I cannot tell you what was in them.

Later Charles became Richard's pupil, but this gradually changed and Richard was induced to take part in Charles's Bible readings and religious services, in which Charles was the leader—probably the clergyman. All this grew out of his relation to one of the hostel staff who intended to become a clergyman.

Marsenland, however, did not appear until Richard developed a calf love (a 'crush') on one of the teachers at school. Marsenland, we were told, was full of awful things, but none of them were dangerous because he, Richard, had so much magic to throw at them. He was 'all magic' because he was 'pink'. Marsenland became a definite place and he made a map of it, which we shall now consider.

The name Marsenland has two roots, one from the name of a grocer's shop (Marsden) near the hostel, to which he used to go on errands for the matron (he bought food there); the other comes from a common interest he had with Charles in Greek and Roman myths—the word contains the name of the god of war. Taken as a whole, then, he is taking up his conflicts over feeding and excreting which, in a general sense, means taking things in (the shop) and putting them out (war). This then belongs to that period when boundaries and the experience of what is me, and not-me develops and when body-imagery begins to emerge. In Richard's case this body-imagery was abstracted into a map, which we may assume to be a magical means of controlling parts of the world. Much of the magic was not depicted in this map for he said that the whole land was full of giants, ghosts and witches. These absorbed him sufficiently for him to pay little attention to ordinary reality. How far his lack of reality could go is illustrated by the following incident. On one occasion he and another boy, with whom he was engaged in earnest conversation, received some rough treatment by the other boys in the hostel: they were tied up with string and thrown into a bed of nettles. When the couple were found, Richard was talking to the other boy; he did not appear at all upset and remarked that he found the nettles 'warming'.

The occasional collapse of his world was expressed when he danced about, made loud noises and fell on the floor; then everything had gone to pieces 'once and for all'.

Following the title of the map was the phrase 'Sheet 23'. This means that it was an Ordnance Survey map; it was not a child's construction but had a grown-up meaning and so represented his denial of being a child.

The map was open on each side, i.e. there were no boundaries to it. I think the town at the top lefthand corner, Marseton, gives further emphasis to the conflict area that is in evidence in the words below it. The map was drawn when the happy days of making worlds was over, when Richard and Charles were fighting over which was the 'true world'. I cannot describe the details of their conflict because it was conducted in private, but there were indications of it in the map. Thus Lighton was named four times: 'Sparfews' was a derogatory epithet and was equated with a different, a later, spelling to which the epithet 'Doonies' was added and underlined. 'Doonies' meant 'lunatic' so his opinion of Lighton was very low. Then it was also an inferno and Lighton Infernae was emphasized by being written in capitals, covering a large area. Below this was the Marsenish empire with a special Marsenish sign attached to it to represent the parts of Charles's world that had been taken over but not assimilated. Richard's name occurred in the middle of 'Lighton Sparfews or Lighton Doonies', suggesting that this was where he asserted himself. Laneytown, below, near the Marsenish empire, was a condensation and contained part of his surname.

Charles's influence was felt elsewhere. Woodbine Sea on the right referred to the happiest times the two boys had together: they played for hours at a time, mapping out the garden according to the names of cigarettes—Woodbines were then the cheapest cigarettes that could be bought and were probably smoked in secret by the older boys in the hostel.

In one other area Charles's influence was represented and there was no boundary line between it and the other areas. 'Yippi-today' and 'tomatown Tommorow of todaytown' was entirely Charles's phraseology, if you cut off the addition of 'town'. These phrases would be used when Charles was in particularly good spirits. The Marsen river connected Marseton with Fightarse, two centres of aggression ('Arse' is the elder boy's name for the anus and buttocks). The river ran close to Fartown and Shitown, of which the names thinly concealed that they were the places for passing flatus and faeces.

Near the mouth of the river Marsen, which is near Fightarse —a linkage between mouth and anus, which might have been expected—was the island of Lars Porsena, which had a special Marsenish mark. Porsena was emphasized in two ways: there was the R. Porsena and there was Porsenathorpe. Richard was familiar with the poem *Lars Porsena* and I think it is safe to assume that this is a reference to the poem.

Lars Porsena of Cruseum by the nine gods he swore
That the great house of Tarquin should suffer wrong
No more, by the nine gods he swore it and named . . .
Day, East and West and South and North his messengers
Ride forth to summon his array . . .

The mouth of the river Porsena had signs of both aggression and ambivalence. There was the island of Marseton, presumably a centre of war; it had also a marsh on it. At the opening, perhaps on the island, were 'Crucifixion' and Crusetown. The crucifixion is at once a horror and a redeeming symbol, as we had at the mouth of the Marsen.

The islands were enclosed areas; there were others, about some of which I can say little or nothing. Carnetland might have been a bit of Charles's world, incorporated and separated off. Tallamclimeshire meant nothing to me, but it was marked with the Marsenish sign and so was probably significant. Godle Sea, being close to the centres of anal activity, would suggest omnipotence. The sea had an outlet, a river that goes to the boundary of Lighton and Tallamclimeshire; and since we know of his interest in urine, this would locate the physical area to which the omnipotent fantasy was moving.

The Marsen Desert might suggest an area of depression, it was, however, close to an oasis, so that if this was an area of depression it was not very serious. Akinshire was perhaps another area of omnipotence.

Duddleby Volcano, almost exactly in the centre of the map, was dangerous and it is related to the schoolmaster with a name like that of the volcano. The master had a violent explosive temper—he 'blows up'. Fattieshire, Fattieland, Bulcote and Skinnietown seemed to contain opposites, but Fatty was, in reality, a boy of great violence as the association Bull-cote indicated. There remains 'gearboxland'. This was part of a secret sexual joke about the schoolmistress I have already referred to. Here he combined with Charles in making jokes and bus games; the teacher came into it since she had a bus service —the bus services were complex and were all written down on lavatory paper. Gabltown referred to the amount of talk that went on and possibly to the teaching of the schoolmistress. The island, Feasern, referred to a hostel visited by the boys, and had a Marsenish sign on it.

Taken as a whole, the encircled areas were all significant because they referred either to experiences from the everyday life of Richard, or to fantasies containing conflicts.

The group of names at the top right area had pleasant associations; they related to places he had been to on outings. In view of what I have said, it is interesting that Albytown seems to refer to a boy who was faecally incontinent, though there did not seem to be any special outer relationship to this boy, i.e. he was not a friend. Below in the middle is 'Neverfield Tijoyce', which meant the place where he went to church. I have no clue to Ferguson, but Carlham is like the name of a place near the hostel. Bibbleton is where King Richard's palace is located; he used only his Christian name. He was king of the whole domain. There was a good deal about Bibbleton and he wrote down how it came into being: 'Well, I have some Marsenish history to tell you. To go on, I have a land of my own called Marsenland. I am the king of it. There is a boy who is a magician in Marsenland whose name is Holly Bibble. My

179

country is Woodbineshire, which Charles and me share. Just a little south is Woodbine city. I have a little private den under the ground which is sheltered by fir trees. In the continent of Marsenland there is a desert where many cannibals live. Holly Bibble himself was a good cannibal. When he heard what that witch had done to Rupert he took her to the gallows and torchered her. When she was dead Holly Bibble took her with him and he waved his hand and said 'Bibbleton appear, please', and immediately it appeared. Then he scraped the flesh off her, he cooked it and he ate it.

'In his house he had a big dungeon where he kept many skeletons and ghosts. Then he took the skeleton of the witch down the dungeon and burnt parts of her body. Next door to him lived the king of the ghosts name Cheriselum who helped him in many ways. In Bibbleton there is a haunted castle which had 15 wicked ghosts in it. He feasted fifteen days on them. Holly Bibble, Cheriselum and me built me a palace.'

The following Bible references further fill out for us the picture of Richard's world system. They were written out by him and actually addressed to the religious member of the staff.

THE BIBLE TEXT BOOK

(This is transcribed exactly as written by Richard)

To

Name: Mr. Henry Jones

Address: The House

1. I am no more worthy to be called thy son, make me as one of they hired servants. St. Luke, Ch. 15, v. 19.
2. He that smiteth a man so that he die shall surely be put to death. Exodus, Ch. 21, v. 12.
3. Six days shalt thou labour and do all thy work. Exodus, Ch. 20, v. 9.
4. I am the true vine and my father is the husbandman. St. John, Ch.15, v.1.
5. In the beginning God created the heaven and earth. Genesis, Ch. 1, v. 1.

6. Be not overcome of evil, but overcome evil with good. Romans, Ch. 12, v. 21.

7. Then Pilate therefore took Jesus, and scourged him. St. John, Ch. 19, v. 1.

8. And Pilate wrote a title and put it on the cross and the writing was JESUS OF NAZARETH THE KING OF THE JEWS. St. John, Ch. 19, v. 19.

9. If thou therefore wilt worship me all shall be thine. St. Luke, Ch. 4, v. 7.

10. And the husbandmen took their servants, and beat one, and killed another and stoned another. St. Matthew, Ch. 22, v. 35.

11. Blessed are the pure in heart for they shall see God. St. Matthew Ch. 5, v. 7.

12. Give us this day our daily bread. St. Matthew Ch. 6, v. 11.

13. Grace be with all them that love our Lord Jesus Christ in sincerity. Ephesians, Ch. 6, v. 24.

14. He destroyed their vines with hail and their sycamore trees with frost. Psalms, 72, v. 47.

15. I have gone astray like a lost sheep, seek thy servant for I do not forget thy commandments. Psalms 11, e. 176.

16. Moses said 'Honour thy father and thy mother and Whoso curseth father or mother let him die the death. St. Mark, Ch. 7, v. 10.

17. Trust ye in the Lord for ever, for in the Lord Jehovah is everlasting strength. ISAIAH, Ch. 26, v. 4.

18. And the fish that is in the river shall die and the river shall stink and the Egyptians shall lothe to drink the water of the river. Exodus, Ch. 7, v. 18.

19. Thus the heavens and the earth were finished and all the host of them. Genesis, Ch. 2, v. 1.

20. Of the tribe of Ephrain Oshea the son of Nun. NUMBERS, Ch. 13, v. 8.

21. These words which I command thee this day shall be in thine heart. DEUTERONOMY, Ch. 6, v. 6.

22. The burden which Habakkuk the prophet did see. HABAKKUK, Ch. 1, v. 1.

23. At midnight there was a cry made Behold the bridegroom cometh go ye out to meet him. ST. MATTHEW, Ch. 25, v. 6.

24. So they went and made the sepulchre sure sealing the stone and setting a watch. ST. MATTHEW, Ch. 27, v. 66.

There is only one further remark I want to make about the world. Eventually there was much more conflict between Richard and Charles, which centred on the question of whose world was true; the collaboration between them became less and less friendly. In the end it was agreed that a long wall was to be built between the two worlds so that no further conflicts could occur.

From what I have said, it can be seen how the places were connected indirectly to people in the outer world, but it was at the same time magical and was an attempt to control the objects in the outer world by magical means. In order to control as much of it as possible, all is taken into the scheme, which was expressed most significantly in the fact that Holly Bibble was a cannibal. It will be apparent here how much the oral schema had become elaborated and how many diverse processes had become associated with it, and at the same time how near at hand the oral ingestion remained in the cannibalism.

I think we can see here how Piaget's processes of assimilation and accommodation worked together with their affective correlates, projection and introjection. The inner processes were indeed accommodated to the outer, but the greater emphasis was on the assimilation, so that the 'inner' processes were enormously developed at the expense of the outer and there was, while this process was active, extremely little effort at adaptation to outer demands. It must be remembered, however, that this world-making was in Richard's spare time and it was allowed to develop as part of the policy we had adopted in running the hostel, because there was such a good matron; it could not have been done without her. At school, Richard was becoming more and more successful and in fact in the end he won a scholarship.

Perhaps the clearest references to his own self lay in his relation to the excretory processes, to his own name and to his being kind; but the whole map is really ultimately of himself and of the processes he was able to experience.

The map could be conceived as representing a coherent dynamic structure in which various parts had been separated off and enclosed because of their dangerous possibilities. The Duddleton Volcano, for instance, was obviously dangerous. The Lars Porsena island contained the idea of righting wrongs, part of which may be said to have started in the Porsena River; and then there was an outpost at Porsenathorpe, though it looks as if the main assault was held in abeyance.

Bibbleton was not marked off, even though a similar theme is found in it—the goodness and creativeness of God and the cruelty of man. Bibbleton was not marked off because in its biblical aspect it is related to the religious member of the staff to whom the biblical quotations were in fact addressed, as I have mentioned above.

It is difficult to make relations with children of this sort unless you first know where they are in their own psyche. But it is not possible to know unless they can tell you or you can spot by inference where they are. To some areas there is free access, and if one can get there it is not so difficult to find out more about some other areas, but the guarded areas are very difficult; one may get a hint of them but one cannot get into them, yet these are the most important ones.

There is not much ego in all this. There is a hint of it in the boy's name and perhaps in 'Akingshire'—but as king he is omnipotent and hence more of a self than an ego. This means he had not at that time much organized consciousness to work with.

Yet this boy developed successfully in the end. A pointer to this is, I think, in the Lars Porsena theme in which wrongs were righted, to a lesser extent in the emergence of Bibbleton, and also in his reaction against Charles's world. These may be regarded as the positive centres representing foci from which recovery was to prove possible.

Further Notes on Charles

This child's early development was difficult. His parents' relationship was bad and divorce proceedings were under way when he was four. At his birth his mother had 'kidney trouble', presumably a toxaemia of pregnancy, though she had enough milk to feed him for three months. He was very slow in walking and talking; he was thought to have something wrong with his legs for he did not get on to his feet till he was three years of age.

When he started going to school, at five years old, he made sudden unprovoked attacks on other children and was always getting 'excited and uncontrolled'. In consequence the head teacher asked for him to be removed and he eventually found his way to the hostel. The mother particularly commented that, though the head teacher could not keep him, she was particularly attached to Charles.

His mother brought him and quite often came back to the hostel; it was from her that this information was obtained. She had some interesting observations, for instance that if he 'shuts his mind it is useless to try and get him back'. She also said he was terrified of the lavatory and could not use the one that flushes because he was afraid he would fall into it, therefore he always used the potty. There was open sex play with little boys and girls and he would keep asking his mother to masturbate him. It would seem that his penis was particularly important because it was small and the testicles were not descended.

In the hostel he soon showed how much he was in a world of his own making, because it was only in very restricted periods that he would conform to hostel routines and handling. He showed a love of and a good command of words, and spent much time making up a running commentary on the wireless itself. He was very much interested in money and would make financial appeals for surprising yet deserving causes, such as the 'starving cats of Europe'. He had, like many of these children, a special love for animals; he adopted a kitten and regularly took her to bed with him.

He was one of the smaller boys in the hostel and he appreciated the danger of attacking others. He dealt with the roughness of the bigger boys by a combination of asserting that he was a grown-up and so not to be attacked, and of abuse combined with screams for help. There was also a magic wand and a piece of paper that he waved about as a defence. He regularly kept near a grown-up, asserting that he was 'a case' or 'I am the only case in the hostel that has to be with a grown-up'.

His sleep was disturbed and he said: 'I hate the nights—don't let me dream. I'd like it to be one long day', and he would ask paradoxically: 'Will you get me to sleep?' This sleep disturbance gradually passed.

He soon revealed that he had an imaginary companion, 'Be

Ure', a gnome, who owned houses and palaces which he knew exactly how to get to. It was this gnome that was at the back of his not complying with the very reasonable and limited restrictions that were imposed on him in the hostel. At times he would be in 'Be Ure's' and land not in the hostel at all.

A great deal of his fantasy was incomprehensible so that, whereas he could be treated as 'Be Ure' and then would comply with requests or other suitable approaches, when he was in the incomprehensible spheres nobody knew how to treat him.

Gradually he developed an imaginary family, the 'Stones', and they had a language of their own. Whether he understood it or not was uncertain because if he did know what it all meant he kept it secret. Most probably he understood but little of their language.

Interestingly enough, he had a very good memory for objective events and, even in his most incomprehensible times, he would suddenly take the hostel staff to task if they made a factual mistake. He also knew the difference between the reality of fantasy and that of the external world. This is the sort of conversation that could take place when he was rational.

Charles:	Do we go to God every night when we go to sleep?
Miss Paull:	Not exactly—at least some people might think of it like that, but I think we go into our dream world—the other side of us.
Charles:	As we are going to sleep does the real-life world go away and the dream world come?
Miss Paull:	Yes; which world do you like best?
Charles:	The real-life world, because the dream world isn't real—nothing in our dreams is real.
Miss Paull:	I think it is just as real, in another way, as what you call our real-life world—one is the light world and the other our shadow world—the other side of us.
Charles:	If you saw an exercise book in your dreams, you wouldn't have it when you woke up.
Miss Paull:	No, but if you bought an exercise book at Mr. Wickham's, you wouldn't have it in your dream world. But if you had an idea in your dreams you might still keep it in your real world.

Charles: What we think about in the real world makes us dream something similar to it. I think the real world and the dream get muddled up sometimes, don't you? Miss Paull, do you think the real world might take the place of the dream world sometimes, and the dream world the place of the real world? The dark world would be light then and the light world would be dark.

Miss Paull: Yes, I think that might happen.

And here is a conversation about a dream:

Charles: Miss Paull, I had a dream last night about my Mummy coming to see me.

Miss Paull: What did you do when she was here?

Charles: We went for a walk by the river, and I dreamt that I was nearly falling down over the bank all the time. And once when I nearly fell over and I looked up for my Mummy, she was lost in the forest.

Miss Paull: What did you do then?

Charles: I was a bit frightened, and then Harry Morrison came and showed me the way; he took me down a dark place, and then we just had to go along a little bit of road and we came home to this house and Mr. Craven was standing in the doorway, and I went in by him and as I was standing there I woke up. Why do you think I dreamt about that, Miss Paull?

Miss Paull: Perhaps you had been thinking about your Mother coming here for her holiday and how you would take her out by the river.

Charles: No, I don't think so; what do you think it means, Miss Paull?

Miss Paull: Well, what I think it might mean is this: that when in your dream you were walking by your Mother and falling down, that is as you used to be at home when you were afraid to do anything without your Mother and hardly ever dared to leave her, even to go to the lavatory. Then when she was lost in the dream that was because you thought you would like to do something on your own, so you lost her; but at first you were still rather frightened so Harry came to help you find your way, and he was the first picture in your mind of the boy you would like to be—a boy who was quiet and gentle, but knew his way about alone, and was not afraid. When he took you home, and Mr. Craven was on the doorstep, that was the man that you will be when you grow up. How does that seem to you?

Charles: I don't know . . . I was rather frightened when my Mummy had left me.

Miss Paull: Yes, and so you were when your Mother brought you here and left you, but now you can do lots of things for yourself and you are not frightened.

Charles: (laughing) I could hardly do anything without my Mummy, I could hardly cut out. (He was cutting out advertisements and maps from a newspaper while talking).

Miss Paull: You wouldn't have dared to cut out and make all those holes in the paper.

Charles: Why wouldn't I? Would the holes have frightened me? I am not frightened now. I only have to put my hand in the holes and I can feel the hard floor underneath.

Miss Paull: That's because you are boss of the scissors and paper now, and you know you can make them do what you want.

Charles: (laughing with intense satisfaction) I am boss of the scissors (waving them and shouting). You have to obey me.

All this insight was periodic. Alongside it went the development of a new family, the 'Tin' family, who were very much regimented and then after three months he announced that there was a land of Lighton. It was this land and his preoccupation with it that led to the other boys starting worlds and to the emergence of Marsenland, which Richard developed. As we have seen, Charles acted at first as initiator.

This land and its contents became a source of considerable irritation to the hostel staff, but I used to visit and try to make them keep it going, for like Richard he was beginning to adapt at school, to which it would at first have been fruitless to send him.

My efforts were, however, only partially successful and pressure was put upon him to give up his inner world so that one day, in order to please the staff, he renounced it. This was heralded with enthusiasm by some of the staff, but I could not feel so sure myself.

The result was for a time gratifying, but it did not last. The fantasy started seeping back in indirect ways, though he pretended that it was absent. In the end the matron, at my instigation, resuscitated it and he made a map of it. This differed from Marsenland in revealing ways. A glance at it shows it to be much less organized than Marsenland and though some of the words are recognizable, i.e. Woodbine, Th(e) Marsen Sea, and while others could perhaps be dissected, i.e. Clun Bush Town, Shirtutnam, a considerable group seemed to make no sense at all i.e. St6w or Uee. Whatever secret sense these 'incomprehensible' words may have made, they are different from those in Richard's world in that they cannot be understood by those in the environment; if they are adapted then they are designed for inner not outer requirements. The result is much more obscure and confusing; this, we may surmise, is why Richard developed resistances to it and added derogatory epithets. Another clear difference is that there does not seem to be any division into good and bad areas and it is far less possible to see purposive trends.

The lack of clear structure, the degree of confusion, the obscure sense and the absence of dynamic balance all suggest a less good prognosis for Charles than for Richard. Indeed, though Charles went on improving while in the special hostel, so that his external adaptation became reasonably good, the closure of the hostel resulted in a regression and he was eventually admitted to a mental hospital; he has not recovered.

ALAN

Introduction

Any patient puzzles his analyst from time to time. Alan did so more than most: he was the first case of childhood psychosis that I had studied in detail, so I learned a great deal from him.

Except for the history, I have arranged the material in the

order in which it emerged. I started by using analytic method in the first interview so no formal history was then taken; instead, it accumulated during the treatment. I have therefore departed from the usual practice: the history, as Alan's parents conceived and presented it piecemeal to the social worker, will be found at the end. It is there considered in relation to matter collected at other hospitals where Alan attended, and analysed in the light of material I obtained from him.

Alan was referred in September 1959 by Dr B. as 'pre-psychotic', or possibly a case of childhood schizophrenia, whose parents were keen for treatment; they were indeed well motivated and, as the subsequent events showed, their family life was good, in the sense that they combined well over the children, especially Alan. I had previously worked in therapy with cases of this kind but had not had the opportunity of seeing one three times a week, so here was an opportunity that I had been looking for; I was keen to start therapy.

I had been given the following information before the first interview by Dr B. Alan's parents had sought psychiatric help when he was four years old from Dr A. and he had attended hospital X for two years, during which he had received 'play therapy'. Since his main symptoms had remained unchanged and his adaptation at school and at home continued to present serious problems and as he scored low in I.Q. tests given at a two-year interval, placement in a special school had at last been recommended by psychiatrist A. Dissatisfied, Alan's parents then sought a second opinion, and it was then that the diagnosis of infantile schizophrenia was made by Dr B. and this was accepted by them.

One striking feature of Alan's report was that the test at hospital Y revealed an unaccountable alteration in his I.Q.: it had risen from 82 to 105 or 110. All the tests had been given by reliable psychologists, so the change could not be put down to faulty testing techniques.*

* Alan was first tested when four years and two months old; he then achieved an I.Q. of 82 on the Merrill-Palmer scale (C.A. 50 months; M.A. 36 months). The report stated that 'he did not seem to be using his potentiality to the full' and so he was tested again at five years and eleven months. His M.A. was then five years and two months, giving an I.Q. of 87. The psychologist appended a note: 'This (I.Q.) contains a high rote memory success, without which the I.Q. would be 82, i.e. very little change from last time'. It was this report that I had seen before the interview, hence the figure 82 in my text. There seems to be an error in the note, for the first I.Q. was 72 and this would mean a significant rise on the second test. The full reports are added in the appendix.

As to his education: Alan's parents had succeeded in placing him in a primary school, and it turned out that they had been particularly fortunate. Alan was not ready for much formal education but his class teacher gave him unusual freedom to move about and even go out of the classroom during lessons; he became interested in Alan and noticed that if allowed to behave in this way the child picked up information and made original comments that engaged the teacher's interest. There was no question of his being asked to leave school and it seemed probable that if treatment was successful his behaviour and capacity to learn would improve.

First Interview

With this information in mind I approached the first interview. During it I hoped to find out whether I could make a relationship with Alan; in particular I wanted to know whether he could form a transference and whether a therapeutic alliance could be established. I was therefore particularly interested to observe his response to any interpretations I might succeed in making.

The first interview—though none of the later ones—was tape-recorded, so essential verbal content can be given in some detail; I shall add descriptions of bits of play to make the verbal record understandable. I shall also give, where interpretation seems difficult to follow, some account of the mental processes that went on in my own mind. This does not mean that I thought consciously along the lines I shall indicate—because my main attention was focused on Alan—but rather that what I record will give the background of half or truly unconscious thoughts that went on in my mind. An alternative would be to construct a theory of the interpretations, but this would give a misleading picture: an analyst has theories in his mind and sometimes they are used as such. It is only when they are, so to speak, in his bones and represent a group of affective experiences with patients in the past that they are of much use. With a patient abstract theoretical thinking is next to impossible because the analyst's affects are too much engaged with his patient.

My objective in writing out this first interview in such detail is not only to illustrate first-interview technique and to introduce Alan but also to give an impression of what Alan's therapy was like.

The interview is a special one in being the first, but it contains many features of any interview and in particular the dialectic nature of the processes that went on then and continued later. In later interviews I usually intervened much less, because Alan's anxieties were not so great and did not urgently need my understanding. In addition there was usually more time to test my ideas before communicating them. Sometimes, when the meaning of his play became very clear, and the verbal dialectic was going well and everything I saw was responded to verbally, I made a good many more interventions than are described in this first interview.

In this interview there was a background of consistency in my understanding based on the relation between Alan and his mother. This contrasts with the otherwise varying activities and statements by him. I have made no attempt to gloss over this disparity and consequently the reader may feel that I was trying to force order on to a muddle that really was truly there. This impression would be justified if I had not been ready to withdraw or alter my understanding in the light of more information and also if I had thought of my interpretations as more than tentative. It is usually after detailed and often long study of a child that interpretations gain a reliability that they cannot have in the setting of a single interview.

Looked at in the light of my later knowledge of Alan, some of my interpretations contained errors, especially my assumption that he would understand the idea of having something— a thought or feeling—inside him; I shall comment on this later. It was important, however, that in spite of these faults there was no lack of capacity on his part to relate, and it was this that I was mainly aiming to test.

When I first met Alan he seemed rather small for a six-year-old, with a pale face and dark hair. He came with me from the waiting-room, where his family was assembled, but developed a dreamy abstracted look. It is very difficult to give a picture of him as a person in this interview because of the changes in mood that took place: first of all he looked dreamy and dissociated, perhaps a schizoid or possibly a schizophrenic child, but later he suddenly changed to a decisive aggressive impulsive person. Though this changeability was not so characteristic of him later on in therapy, because a particular mood tended to predominate in any particular interview (and indeed over quite long periods of time), this first interview was especially significant in suggesting that his personality split up rather easily, so that he presented bits of himself unrelated to the rest of him. It may be because of this state that he is so difficult to describe: he seems to be several persons rather than one, and this suggested that there was no core to his personality and that I would be compelled to pay attention to any part of him that happened to be functioning at any particular time.

Once in the play-room, where the psychiatric social worker was sitting in a chair, he went to the window and peered down the main road, which could easily be seen, was full of traffic and stretched away into the distance. I asked him whether he was looking for something outside. Without replying he picked up a toy and put it in his mouth; then he made a vague remark about somebody being a long way outside the window. As the behaviour was related to his leaving his mother, I said:

Dr F.: When you come in here, it feels like your mummy is a long, long way away, miles and miles away; and you're afraid you won't be able to see her again. You'd like to have her inside your mouth and then she couldn't get away. And you'd be happy?

Alan: I wouldn't. (very emphatically).

Dr F.: (disconcerted): You wouldn't because there's something inside* you that would want to?

Alan: No (again he was very emphatic).

Dr F.: (still put out): That's a good thing. I thought you might have something inside you that felt like that ... but you want me to think you're good. (At this point the dreamy, abstracted look returned.) So I said, She's a long way away again—you feel she's gone away—going to leave you—that must be a horrid feeling—but your mummy would never really do that, would she?

Alan: Yes, she would.

---

* Viewing this episode in the light of what I came to know about Alan's 'inner world', the word 'inside' was probably inappropriate and 'a bit of yourself' would in retrospect have been better. I do not think I could have known this at the time.

Dr F.: She didn't look to me the sort of mummy who would go away and leave you. Perhaps she *has* done it; didn't you go to hospital before?

Alan: Why, why do we go to hospital? (Later, after I enquired about its name, and whether he found my room like the other one, he reiterated in a desperate questioning voice, 'Why? Why?')

Dr F.: (meditating): Why? Yes, indeed.

Alan: I think she'll go too far away and I won't be able to get to her. (Here I wondered whether this confirmed my first interpretation or whether he was identifying himself with it.)

Dr F.: Wouldn't she want you to get to her? She feels like that, does she . . . ? She's got that baby there (i.e. in the waiting-room), hasn't she, and when you go out (of the waiting-room) it makes a difference—mummy's a long way away, mummy's with the baby?

Alan: Yes (followed by mumbles).

This marks the end of the first part of the interview; after it Alan's behaviour changed. His startling and emphatic style of expression was rather characteristic but, though he repudiated my interpretations—or rather a part of them, on the whole he recognized them as relevant. As a result, his distrust of his mother, and by inference of me too, became clear. Distrust of her is related to going to hospital and also to her being with the baby.

There are features of my interpretations that gave me cause for reflection: they indicated the beginning of a counter-transference, which was in part helpful but also was one that could lead to more or less serious difficulties.

This is not the place to dilate upon this subject, but it is noteworthy that Alan consistently provoked those in his environment to irrational estimates of him. Thus my countertrans-ference can be thought of as reflecting a general state of affairs. His parents' and his school-teacher's feeling about him was basically positive, and so I was justified in my estimate; but this carried with it other features, which I thought of with sceptical interest. I have said that I was disconcerted by his emphatic denials; I had not expected anything so organized from a child who was so dreamy and remote. Yet I might have expected a denial, for the idea that led to my interpretation was as follows: I was drawing on other experiences with children which indicated that dreamy far-away feelings had been associated with that of being swallowed up, and this implied a mouth; when he put an object in his I connected the two. Since the feeling of being swallowed can be a negation of swallowing, my interpretation followed quite easily. Alan's denial therefore may have contained the denial left out of my communication: I was—in short—formulating the affect that was denied. The phrase 'and you would be happy' seems to have been added because of my own distress at seeing Alan in such a state; in some part of me I could not bear it and wished he would be happy; thus there was evidence of unconscious denial on my part.

The second interpretation, though on the right lines, provides further food for reflection, especially because of the rather defiant emphasis in my tone of voice, which I have not indicated in my description. Again there was an emphatic 'No' from Alan and my next remarks covered hesitation and uncertainty. This can be shown in the verbal content: there was no need to say 'That's a good thing' nor to explain 'I thought you might have something inside you that felt like that'. Nevertheless the overall content of my intervention was still relevant and, in spite of my countertransference, I felt confident enough to enquire about his mother; once again he was emphatic, but this time about her. The view of his mother that Alan was giving here probably contained a reference to a traumatic event that I did not know of at the time. Alan became inaccessible to his mother two months after his younger brother was born: the baby developed pyloric stenosis and she went into hospital with him and this necessitated leaving Alan with his father (for further details cf. infra p. 249).

Returning to the interview record: the change in Alan's mood was reflected in his look; it was no longer distraught but alive and 'on the spot'. He became interested in the sand-tray, which had in it some water and a bucket. He said something indistinctly that I thought was a communication:

Dr F.: What? I didn't hear that; will you tell me again?
Alan: . . . sand in there . . . (i.e. in a bucket that was available. I reflected that he might be using the bucket to

represent his mother, or part of her; but he next asked a question, indicating that his thoughts were moving in a different direction).

Alan: What is it meant for? What is the sand meant for? (After this he moved over to the sink, which was too high for him to reach the tap.)

Dr F.: Would you like to put some water in it and fill it up? (I lifted him up and put a chair for him to stand on; he then used the water from the tap and put it in a pot.)

Alan: I've got sand in it. (He hesitates and looks anxious.)

Dr F.: Well, that would be all right, wouldn't it? (Reflectively). You have sand in playgrounds, don't you? Down by the sea you have sand. Or do you have sand at home?

Alan: Not at home . . . (and he burst out laughing and denied it again).

Dr F.: You seem to have lots of funny thoughts about what people are like inside . . . Could you tell me what your thoughts are—what makes you laugh? What have you seen that's funny?
(Alan then came and sat on my lap and put his cheek against mine in a rather sensual loving way, then he rubbed his nose against mine). I said: 'Oh, that was your joke was it, rubbing noses?' Next he tried to push my mouth open with his fingers. 'Ah! You want to look to see what's inside my mouth.'

Alan: You are funny!

Dr F.: I'm such a funny man! (He pinched my nose with his fingers and tried to twist it round.) You want to screw it off? What do you want my nose for? To go smelling about with? (He then mouthed it and alternated this activity with putting his thumb in his mouth. Then followed some inaudible remarks. He got off my lap and started to look inside other objects—a box, a cupboard that was there; he seemed interested, yet afraid.)

Dr F.: You want to look inside them?

Alan: What's in them?

Dr F.: What do you think is inside them?

Alan: I don't know.

Dr F.: You wouldn't be afraid to look, would you? (He laughed.) It would be such a funny thing; what would happen?

Alan: I don't know, but I might touch it.

Dr F.: Would you dare? What would happen?

Alan: It might bite me.

Dr F.: Would it bite you? Have you got a naughty mouth that wants to bite people?

(Alan laughed and there followed a lot of active play; he looked inside a box and found a tiny baby.)

Dr F.: A baby . . . perhaps you were expecting a baby inside there. (There followed a change in activity.)

Alan: Where's the bucket . . . ? Ooh, this is tight . . . look, there's water in the sand.

(By now I was sure he was accessible and responded to interpretations, in other words, analytic treatment was worth starting—indeed, it had already begun.)

Dr F.: I'm going to fetch your mummy now, or would you like to fetch her? Shall I fetch her?

Alan: What for?

Dr F.: Well, we are going to have a talk about you. Perhaps you wouldn't like her to come and talk about you.

Alan: Ooh, there's the water. (Referring to the sink with a tap over it.)

Dr F.: Well, I'll fetch your mummy and you can play with the water. . . .

It seemed suitable to introduce Alan's mother at this point because he had made a relation to the objects in the room, which suggested that he was going to start playing.

I did not understand the remark about water then, but, from what transpired, it contained aggressive intent. I went out to the waiting-room and brought Alan's mother into the play-room. She greeted Alan with 'Oh darling, what are you doing?', referring to his play, which was by now quite active. Alan took no notice and, having said this, she sat down.

I started by looking over the notes from Dr B. and said that he had told me quite a lot about Alan and that I wanted to confirm that she and her husband were agreeable to the proposed treatment.

At this point, Alan exclaimed (presumably with reference to his play, to which I was not paying attention): 'Get them out quickly!' This came before mother could reply to my communication to her: 'Yes, fairly regularly.' Again Alan interjected: 'Yes, get them out quickly or they will drown.' This was the last time he made any remark while mother and I were talking and, as it was then that I introduced the subject of treatment, I reflected that his remarks might be connected with it.

Mother and I went on to work out the times at which she could bring Alan and I said treatment could start at once. Mother replied, 'Oh good; I'm very pleased to hear that'. Next, I asked her whether she would tell me something of what she felt was the matter with Alan. My object here was to give Alan some idea of why his mother thought he should come, having in mind Alan's distraught 'Why, why do we go to hospital?'. She made a characteristic response.

Mother: Well, what is worrying myself and my husband is—
is it all right to speak in front of him?
Dr F.: Well, I expect you will say things that he will know about, won't you? (With this she agreed and went on to speak quite easily.)
Mother: It is his complete lack of being able to get on with people.
(This concerned her, and she amplified this by referring to family relations and especially that he seemed 'wrapped up in his own little world' and had no friends. As a consequence he had not settled down well at school.)

She then went on to talk about the past: she and her husband had thought that having another baby would help, but it had not turned out as they had hoped. Without prompting, she continued talking of the difficulties resulting from Alan being born with talipes. 'Sometimes I think that's the real root of the trouble', she said. 'Probably, in my ignorance, I was much too vigorous and rough, too keen to get the feet right, and did not think enough about the psychological effect'. She had been instructed to massage Alan's feet and apply the splints that had also been prescribed. Alan used to scream and 'when he was a tiny thing he used to pull my hair'. Since then, he had pulled many people's hair, particularly that of children. Later on he saw 'pixies' and remarked that their toes turned up, saying that they were like his.' 'I think', she continued, 'that it did prey on his mind and he is the type who bottles things up . . . he doesn't express his feelings very well and I think he gets rid of his pent-up emotions by his aggressive attitude to people.'*

Through all this Alan's mother expressed her feeling that in behaving as she had done she had harmed her son, had caused his present condition, about which she was guilty—could she not have managed better? This information is over-determined: is mother saying something true about Alan or is her guilt the more important, covering up feelings of hostility towards him? At this point it was important to suspend judgment.

Since she had now given reasons for referral that Alan could appreciate, I started to end the interview with her by introducing the psychiatric social worker and saying she could say more to her later on, and fixed the time of the next interview.

During my conversation with mother, Alan had been playing with water in the sink. When she had gone I went over and watched his activities. He was swishing the water about with his hand, turning the water-tap on and off, pulling out and reinserting the plug, also taking sand out of the sand-tray, carrying it to the sink and dropping it into the water. From time to time he reached down to the bottom of the sink and scooped the sand out with his hands. He kept saying that the tide was rising, and it would soon be washing all over the place. I said; 'It looks as if you wanted to drown your mummy and me while we were talking.' The play became more vigorous, a boat and fish appeared—perhaps, I thought, a reference to mother and me—and there was recurrent concern with the depth of the water.

I asked him whether he remembered his mother doing all those horrid things to his feet. He said 'Yes' and then wanted to give me sand from the bottom: 'There's some sand for you' and this I accepted and said I would keep it safe, because it seemed like a bit of gratitude for my understanding something of what he felt.

Dr F.: I thought your mummy was telling me a lot of the time how she felt she was a nasty mummy, and not a good mummy, and she had babies, and she was nasty to you when she didn't want to be, and how you felt still that she was going to be nasty; so you didn't want to have much to do with her—and you are showing me with

* This was a conclusion she had arrived at during her interviews in Hospital A.

the water how you feel about mummy—and that must
be very nasty . . .

Alan: There's not any sand. (This would suggest that there is
no good object any more—there is no good bit of mummy
left, for in reality there was still plenty of sand.)

Dr F.: You are really doing—when you saw the sand there—
what you would like to do when you found some and
felt it was like my inside . . . You're washing me out—
that's all the bad things inside me, isn't it, that you are
washing away? Like when we talked about the sand,
and you thought it was so funny, and I said the sand
was inside me. You're making me good—aren't you—
with the water—with the good water—washing away
all the bad man—all these bad inside things? (I had
here assumed that because there is no good sand it
had turned bad—The bad things inside.)

Alan: See this . . . in the sink . . . see you don't fall in it.

I was interested in his showing concern about the effect of
his wishes expressed in both thoughts and actions at once. Up
to this time he had been ruthless.

Alan: Yes . . . or you'll be drowned . . . (Suggesting that he
has accepted my earlier interpretation.)

Dr F.: You don't want me to be drowned after all—you think
I'm quite a nice man and will do all right—you don't
want me to disappear and be dead. It's quite changed
from when you first came, hasn't it? When I came into
that room and you thought, 'Oh, I don't like this man—
what's he doing to do to me? And what shall I do to
him, if I'm not careful?' I don't like water put on me,
it's true. (This last sentence referred to a frustrated
impulse of his to throw water at me.)

Alan: Oh, look, you can't see the sand.

Dr F.: And all the bad things have gone away.

Alan: Look, I'm getting out the sand—washing the sand,
getting the sand away—ooh, it is getting a mixture.
Oh look! There's hardly any sand. Oh, you can't see
any sand, can you?

These comments were accompanied with action: when
getting rid of the sand he took the plug out and tried to push

sand on the bottom of the sink down the waste pipe. As he did this vigorously the sand became stirred up making a 'mixture', so obscuring the sand at the bottom ('You can't see any sand'). Thus there was a basis in reality for his symbolic play. Though there is a doubt implied in his last question, his play represented an achievement and provided a suitable note on which to end the interview.

Reviewing it as a whole, there are features of the dialectic that developed which were repeated throughout therapy. His response to what I said could be very direct; there was also his delayed verbal acceptance of my interpretations and there were indirect responses that are difficult to convey. Instead of answering in my idiom he continued with his own, developing his play and his thoughts as if they were not related to mine; if the details of the play had not altered as he heard what I said it might be thought that the dialectic had been interrupted. As his play did alter I learned to take this as an indication that what I said was having an effect and was being assimilated.

It is difficult to substantiate this from the tape-recording only, but I believe I have described sufficient of the play to make sense of the dialogue; if I had done more it would not have helped. What I have not described are the movements, looks, glances and the like, which were so quick and yet so significant. In spite of these omissions, which I do not know how to convey, I hope I have made graphic the experience of mutual understanding between us. It was growing all through this interview: Alan's analysis had begun.

Before describing the main body of it I shall comment on some of his rather striking characteristics. He tended to evoke the interest and emotions of those in his environment; in his therapy it could be felt clearly as a countertransference. He evoked in me the feelings of care, interest and belief in himself, which were his own qualities in a very primitive stage of development.

His behaviour was often crude, violent and outrageous, but, though it evoked anger, it was anger linked with regret at having been angry. His apparent lack of reality sense, and his daring, made him appeal to the half-conscious shadow of grown-up people, but it evoked care at the same time, though he often rejected this.

In addition to the dexterity of his mind, his unusual interests, his surprising and often original remarks, his decisiveness and, as his analysis developed, his capacity for insight fascinated grown-up people near to him, made them have confidence in his future or feel that he was a child with unusual potential.

His parents felt this from early on and it made them reject the unfavourable recommendation of Dr A., which seemed quite justified at the time. Of course this was also denial on their part of the narcissistic injury that Alan's existence represented, but it was not only that, for they thought and reflected about him in a caring and objective way. Furthermore, others experienced him in a similar way. Dr B. was interested and hopeful, and Alan's teacher was willing to allow special freedoms, which meant treating him as an unusual and worthwhile person. It was these characteristics that also made me keen to do all I could for him.

Analytic Therapy

The description of Alan's treatment will be divided up into five overlapping parts, as in a fugue. In each part a particular theme became prominent and dominated the others, which then sank into the background.

SUMMARY OF THE STAGES

In the first part his play was active, restless and manic; as the energy in this worked itself out he developed a ritual framework to his activities—the second part. In the third part a homosexual transference emerged; it was quite short and in the fourth part, also relatively short, he worked over a sadistic primal scene, culminating in his supervision of a good intercourse between 'animal' parents. The last part was mainly structured in terms of 'goodies and baddies'—cowboys and Indians and the like—and reflected his entry into the latency period. Ending may be taken as a short sixth episode and as there was still some work to be done with his environment—especially his school—a seventh, post-analytic, part.

Technique

My attitude and technique, except when physical intervention was necessary, were consistently analytic.

I aimed all the time to elucidate and understand Alan's verbal and motor behaviour with the aim of reaching the root of his conflicts. In the course of my summary of his treatment I shall detail only some of what I said—especially that part of it which proved crucial in my relation to him. But there was, for some of the time, a rather continuous conversation rather like the one I described in the first interview but which is not included in the description. The dialectic led to complications: Alan started competing with me in saying what a particular bit of play meant; he would get in first with what I was going to say, or make rather challenging statements to see what I would do with them. When this happened, I would interpret his feelings of rivalry and his wish to show that I was not necessary to him, or that he was feeling my talk as a threat that he wanted to neutralize by out-doing me.

Interpretation of the meaning of my talk prevented or rather dissolved the danger of my becoming, in his feeling, a persecuting teacher-analyst and it sustained the overall good transference/countertransference relation; this was, during the whole treatment, never seriously in danger of breaking down, but, without consistent attention being paid to it, it might have done so.

There were periods in which I would be talking rather continuously about what he was doing and there would be indications, from changes and developments in his play, that he was taking note of parts of my communications but not of them all. Then it was as if he was primarily enjoying my interest and felt I was concerned for him. Again, there would be times when he took no notice, like a child who thinks that grow-ups go on like that—it is all 'bla bla', not worth taking any notice of. Following these feelings and interpreting them, the first in terms of my words representing a good breast-feed, and the latter like a mother trying to give the breast when he was not hungry but interested in playing, would result in his greater capacity to react more specifically to what I said.

These examples illustrate the need for constant attention to transference manifestations. They could often be arrived at not so much by observation of Alan as by taking note of my countertransference. How an analyst feels about his patient, and this applies especially with children, is an essential clue to the transference; and, in the case of a schizoid child, his

NB

capacity for projective identification is such that the analyst experiences it first and can then make observations that confirm his feeling of what is going on. In each of the examples covering my talk as a whole, there was a period in which I was rather sure that Alan was using me as a feeding mother, but there was for quite a time nothing to indicate whether what I felt was true or false.

The countertransference sometimes led me to make interventions that were premature or incomplete but sometimes strikingly confirmed later on—an example of this will be detailed later (cf. p. 232); but over and over again it made valuable interventions possible, which resistance to it on my part would have prevented. That rather free reliance on countertransference can lead to minor inaccuracies or mistakes seems inevitable, but the advantages of relying upon it greatly outweigh the disadvantages; the mistakes show up, can be worked over and corrected (cf. first interview).

So as not to give the impression that I was verbally active all the time, it is necessary to say that the amount I talked was variable and there were quite long periods, several weeks for instance, when I said very little. This happened when Alan was developing a theme, a story or when, as in Part Three, he was structuring his interviews as a broadcast, with himself as both the announcer and the person making the broadcast. It would not have been difficult to intervene but I did not: to be sure, as the listener to the broadcast, I could not possibly intervene. But a stronger reason still was the fact that the form of his communication needed to be respected, and to interpret its defensive aspects would have been an intrusion that would dislocate rather than foster my analytic aim.

So far I have referred to what I said in general terms. To go into great detail would not, I think, be especially illuminating and I cannot think of a better way than selecting the kinds of activity that were recurrent and characteristic of what I did.

1. There were clarifications of his thought, which was liable to become confused because of its rapidity and the quick switches that he made in it from time to time. I did this without necessarily telling him why the confusion had arisen; indeed, I often did not know myself why his thought had become disorganized at any particular point.

2. On occasion, I put the content of his play into words, thus translating what he did rather than interpreting.
3. *Interpretations:* These were the most important communications. They differ from others in that they contain an inference about an unconscious affect, whether defensive or instinctual. It is usually said that to interpret correctly, the defence against an unconscious content should be analysed first. Looking through Alan's notes, I cannot say that I followed this technique—indeed, it was quite frequently the reverse. I defined the content that was being resisted first and then worked through the defence afterwards. I think, however, that almost all Alan's activities could be taken as a defence against his depression, but the reason for my so thinking will not be given till the history is included in the discussion.

SECTION TWO

The Manic State

In the play-room where I saw Alan, there was a sink with a tap and drain; there was also a moveable sand-tray, two or three buckets, a table and a cupboard with toys in it. There were two comfortable chairs. The floor was covered with linoleum that was not waterproof.

For most of the time I sat in a chair but got up to help Alan if he was in 'technical' difficulties; e.g. if the water tap was too stiff for him to turn on I would help, or if he could not move the sand-tray without jerking it so that the water spilled over.

At first his play was relatively quiet, like the first interview, and I continued talking to him. I did not make many interpretations once the pattern of his play became established, because I found that it was mostly enough to clarify or translate; moreover, his talk was very rapid and the change in ideas so quick that to take up one of them with a view to interpreting would have been like saying things to an absent person. He would, however, take up, deny, confirm or expand my remarks and appreciate that I was taking notice all the time. Interpretations in their proper sense were therefore only occasional and I kept mainly within the imaginative and play idioms that he himself used. In doing so I was influenced by Jung's conceptions and practices, well expressed when, with reference to the psychotic transference, he says: 'The kind of approach must therefore be plastic and symbolical, and itself the outcome of personal experience with unconscious contents "and later" . . . we are best advised to remain within the framework of traditional mythology'. (1946, p. 268).

I did not think much in terms of formal mythological data, though much was included in Alan's idiom and it was within that that I thought. The other influence was the work of Melanie Klein; I would not presume to imagine that I treated children's material as she did, but it was she who made it possible for me to translate 'traditional mythology' into infantile fantasy, which flourished so much in Alan's material, conceived as a basic feature of a child's life.

It was not long before Alan's play became active and excited; it was accompanied by verbal comments, explanations of what was going on and short 'stories' that would switch from one subject to the next. In excited play he used toys but the objective function of the toy had little significance for him; he would use it to represent anything that he wished it to. Sand and toys were used as signs for objects, i.e. not as their nature would suggest. They were often thrown about and always used in a manner that was dictated by his impulses, his fantasy or the logic of his ideas. In a sense he did not play, for there was a desperate content in much of it, which did not correspond with ordinary play. Sand and water were used more than any other materials and he started by carrying water in a bucket from the tap to the sand-tray or sand from the tray to the sink. As time went on, however, he conceived the idea of putting the sand-tray over by the sink; this facilitated transfer of water or sand. In the end he settled mostly on water, with which he would fill up the tray and then make storms by rocking the container.

Though ideas and action were so closely interwoven, it was the ideas that needed close attention for, if the train of thought was not followed and clarified by me when he sometimes could not follow it himself, he would become anxious and tend to act violently, in a disorganized way that was difficult to manage.

His thinking was based largely on analogy. He extracted the common feature of two otherwise very different conceptions, finding sameness in difference. Once this was understood it was not difficult to follow the working of his mind. Thus water represented babies' urine felt by babies to make floods; this was like rain, which was God urinating, so babies were good like God. Rain-urine was dangerous and in crises it would be released as urinary incontinence, which once or twice happened in the interview. God flooded the world to drown people, just as babies imagined they could drown parents and especially mummy. But urine could be good and be drunk like milk; on the other hand, it could be evil and full of poisonous germs, which bring death. So God could be good or bad.

He used the water to make the biggest sea in the world— 'bigger than the Thames or the Atlantic Ocean'. Numerous fantasies were enacted upon it: prominent amongst them were storms and floodings; in contrast, water was also soft and plastic, so it became mother whom he caressed and stroked. It was mother's milk and became an ocean inside babies; he sucked in the water-breast so that he came to possess a 'minnick breast', which could feed an unlimited number of babies and restore damaged parents.

It was also father's milk that was in his genital and which was sucked or ejected into his mother to feed and give pleasure. When he felt that his destructiveness had created a desert, then water would redeem the situation as rain or as a river (of tears). Again, water in a sink would represent the inside of people and have objects that could swim about in it or jump in and out. He gained much satisfaction from looking at what went on, often initiating his account with the word 'Look'.

All these meanings for water were expressed verbally by him and were accompanied by suitable activities, using toys. Sand and Plasticine he also used—only rarely for constructive purposes, however. Mostly they were instruments of aggression for bombing: Plasticine he found useful as a missile.

The mixture of creative ingenuity and the direct naive simplicity of symbolic (analogic) thought, guided by his affect, produced Alan's play and fantasy: it was very impressive. The way in which his thought ran on, and would both follow and inspire very rapid switching from one activity to another, corresponded to quick changes in mood, as in the first interview.

That God was a baby related to the idea of baby Jesus, with which he had been made familiar; that God drowned or destroyed the world with rain which made oceans referred to Noah and the flood. The feeling that violence was 'good' made God being aggressive acceptable, for it was the bad behaviour of the Israelites that made God angry and want to punish them. Sometimes, however, this feeling began to show ambivalence: one day he was using sand and Plasticine to represent poisonous number two (faeces) to attack and poison bad daddy: towards the end he rather regretfully asserted that God made him do it; so it was not surprising to hear him say that God gave him bad thoughts and made him want to do bad things; concurrently he developed a different idea about Jesus, who was naughty: that was why he was crucified.

In this period he could be very incensed if anybody asserted that God was good and, indeed, once had to be removed from Sunday School because he contradicted his teacher, shouting out 'It's not true, God is not good; he is bad' and went on protesting, so that the teacher could not proceed with the lesson and he had to be taken away.

Another interesting idea that he produced later on, when his acute conflicts had become less intense, was that there was a 'fatty God'. He made observations about women, who were called 'fatty', and during the Harvest Festival he shouted, 'Fatty God'. For quite a time after this he talked about 'fatty God', who did bad things to Alan and let Jesus die on the cross.

At this period it was as if Alan was living in a 'mad world', populated by fantastic people and objects. The phrase 'living in a mad world' describes how he experienced it as separate from him and led me to make interpretations based on the idea that the objects were not part of himself, i.e. his ego. Had I embarked on analysing them in terms of inner-world concepts, i.e. that the Minnek sea was inside him or that the desert referred to depressed feelings, it would only have confirmed the idea that I understood nothing, so what I said would not have carried any weight. It is only an adult who could think of his experiences as part of his internal world, for Alan it was a world of imagination and play that he entered when he came into the therapy room and it was always related to objects in the room. Thus he exteriorized conflicts and they seemed like people battling with and loving each other, being adored, cut up or drowned.

Alan's state was essentially manic and was expressed verbally and in action, as in the flight of ideas in the manic disorders of adults. His extremely fluid state of mind gave meaning to the corresponding flood of activity. Among it all, however, there were nuclear themes that were relatively simple:

1. Babies were bad and dangerous because of their excreta. They made oceans that endangered mother by drowning and they threatened her by poisoning; on the other hand, there was baby Jesus, who was essentially good though also naughty.
2. Mother was either good or bad, never both. There was a good mother with a good soft breast who 'rode on a piece of foam' and was his own real good mother and he made up a poem about her:

> 'You can ride home
> On a piece of foam.'

On the other hand, there was a bad threatening magical witch-mother who made poisonous food and was killed by drowning, bombing or other means. Some of the most violent episodes took place in the sink with a boat and a witch in it. To sink the boat and drown the witch was not enough and she had to be pursued to the bottom of the water, which was consequently obscured by the quantity of sand and other objects he threw at her. This made his activity greater because he could not see what she was doing.
3. His relation to father was more personal. After coming to see me, his own father became bad and an enemy and I was adopted as his good father-analyst. The separation of his good from his bad father was reinforced by the physical punishments that his father inflicted from time to time, whereas I did not. He would cause his own father much pain with his explicit refusal to do anything but hate him, and he was not to be mollified. Once his father bought him a book that he wanted, but Alan told him, 'I still don't love you and I never will'.

Besides his personal relationships he developed a variety of interests: in a compass and its four poles, N.S.E.W.; in astronomy and in numbers. These were part of his positive relating to his father, who was interested in such subjects. A little about astronomy and the stars came into the therapy but much more about the compass and the four poles of the world, which were often referred to. Numbers he 'played' with extensively (his father was a statistician). He divided them into little ones, with which he could do sums, addition, subtraction, multiplication and division, and big numbers that could not be used; they were 'magical millions'. None the less, he developed a shorthand for them: thus 6 3 2 meant six millions, three thousands and two hundreds. His preoccupation with size was also expressed in his fantasies of water; there was water in a bucket that could be manipulated and the ocean called the 'Atlantic ocean' or 'Minnek', a term that developed as follows: he was playing with water, 'It's the biggest sea, very big tide made by rain, it's raining in the desert, it's Minnek'. Of the sea he once said 'The sea is very deep and the sky is in it and even if all the sky were in it the sea would be over it'. There was also the river Thames, but this came in less regularly.

Reflections on Alan's Fantasy Life

In this part of his treatment, Alan showed the features of a manic state in a schizoid (some would say schizophrenic) child. It is not my intention to consider its origin till his history has been detailed. But there are features of the symbolism that have interesting implications when considered in relation to the theory of archetypes, which may now be taken up.

Alan's play contained fascinating myth-like material. There was much thought in it, often called omnipotent, because there was little need for the restrictions of reality and free rein could be given to imagination; it is also called magic or mythopeic thinking when exploited in mythology and made into stories like those Alan himself constructed. It is much influenced by primary processes in Freud's sense: the need for immediate and direct discharge of affect, the ready displacement from one object to another and the condensation in the symbols all point in this direction. The primary process, however, does not include word-representations, so evident in Alan's case; furthermore, there is some logical thinking and so it includes secondary processes as well—this combination has sometime been referred to as primary-process thinking. Jung called it undirected thinking and here the idea of playing can be brought in, though this was not Jung's explicit conception of it.

The self and autism

I have already assembled the main significances that water took on for Alan and suggested that the symbolism was constructed by finding 'sameness in difference'; it was this that made the one medium serve so many different purposes. Here I need only provide a reminder by citing a remarkable diversity in the meanings that Alan discovered: on the one hand, it represented extensity and size, as in 'Minnek'; on the other hand, parts of the body, such as babies' urine or mother's soft breast.

The sources of the symbolic images were of three kinds, combined in various ways: 1. Observations of environmental happenings 2. Knowledge gained from books or hearsay. 3. Repressed memories. Each could be observed or reconstructed in Alan's case.

1. Though he lived in London, he had been for holidays by the sea and had been fishing with his family in a boat; then he had been impressed by the waves and their dangerous potential, especially when he heard of people being drowned. He had also been fascinated by the depth of the water and peered down into it; its size also engaged his attention and he wondered about the horizon; finally, he had seen people swimming, though he himself could not do so.

   This leads on to the observations he made and remembered about babies. Here there is little specific information, though he would have seen the way babies' urine is treated as something to be done away with. Further, a baby that is wet cries as if he were hurt or in danger; then mother comes to his aid and removes the wet nappy.

   In other words it may have been an inference that urine was dangerous that fed his fantasies. There may also have been other daily events that were important, though no information was given: bathing, in which the plug-hole of the bath can be centre of excitement and even fear; there might also have been excited swishing about and making waves, playing with boats and other toys and so forth.Then there is the lavatory and the 'flood' of water resulting from pulling the chain, with consequent disappearance of faeces and urine.

2. A second source of material was fairy tales and the Bible, especially the story of the crucifixion and of Noah and the flood; he selected, for special attention, the account of God

making the rain and flooding the earth. Linked with these stories through the idea of the god-baby (baby Jesus) was the notion that a baby's urine makes floods and is dangerous.

3. Finally, there must have been repressed early experiences that can only be inferred by reconstruction: the symbolism may have stemmed from the time when he was a baby; then his urine and faeces were not controllable; the urine might have been felt like a flood and faeces like bombs, which threatened his mother's existence.

There are the evident or possible external or historical sources combined in the play-material. They were selected from a wide range of experiences, as if he were using objects in the world to express his own needs rather than having the events, mental or physical, impressed upon him. He was, indeed, extremely resistant to influence, so this search for sources begs the question of why Alan made so much use of the imagery and experience of water at his disposal. It seems that it was because water could be used and imagined about so easily and proved such an excellent medium through which to exteriorize and express his affects; therefore he found that, in using his mind, he could begin to obtain a measure of control over them.

Alan's use of water in play was determined mainly by his affects, while his need to find representation through objects often led to what can only be called invention, which may have involved hallucination or a sort of revelation. This often looked like primitive but nonetheless creative reflection when he stroked the water and called it mother's soft breast; or it became revelation when the danger of babies' urine was linked to dangerous storms and floods. Then babies became truly omnipotent, as he may have felt as a baby.

The Theory of Archetypes and the Self

Alan's fantasies without doubt contain mythological themes that he combined with personal experience observations and inferences in original ways. The theory of archetypes assumes them to be organizers that select relevant themes from the environment.

From the point of view of the self theory the multiplication of forms points to the predominance of deintegrative processes and I shall now show, by comparing Alan's material with Jung's analysis of alchemy and the myths of the child, that there is evidence of self-representations in his sense.

I was first very much struck by the analogy between the great variety of meanings that Alan gave to water and the use to which alchemists put it. According to them water was a symbol of the *prima materia*, which had a thousand names; these seem to have collected them in much the same way as Alan had and as a result of a mixture of observation, thought, imagination and vision. This is not peculiar to alchemy; indeed, the symbolism of water has one of the widest ramifications in mythology and ethnology. Alchemy seems, however, to be the most relevant because in Jung's theory it was a precursor of individuation initiated by the self. Since I have extended the notion of individuation to infancy and childhood the alchemical analogy appears to me of special interest.

Of course, there are many differences between a child's fantasy and those of an alchemist, but they seem less significant than the similarities and can be accounted for by the additional sources for making fantasies available to alchemists. All of those available to a child would have been available to alchemists but they added a great many more through their chemical or philosophical interests. It is therefore surprising that one can sometimes find quite a number of symbols like Alan's among their texts: here for instance is a list of synonyms. An anonymous writer says: ' . . . the *prima materia* itself consists of composite water—some alchemists put three (waters) together, others two. For myself two species are sufficient: male and female or brother and sister. But they also call the simple water *poison*, quicksilver, cambar, aqua permanens, gum, vinegar, *urine*, *sea water*, *dragon* and *serpent*' (italicised words indicate close analogies with Alan's material) (Jung, 1944, p. 224).

Like Alan, the alchemists included religious imagery as well as exteriorization into matter. According to Jung, they, like Alan, experienced the unconscious through imagery and the proliferating symbolism was enhanced by the possibilities for projection through which image-formation could take place and their interrelations be discovered.

Turning now to another aspect of Jung's work: the parent images often conform to archetypal criteria but the most interesting in the concept of Alan's fantasy is Jung's discussion of the child symbolism that he organized in a special essay: 'The psychology of the child archetype'. There he considered the imagery of myth in relation to his concept of the self as the forerunner of individuation.

The child archetype, Jung says, is predicated in the group of myths that centre round the child as God (Christ, Dionysos, Hermes, Apollo, Pan) or as hero (Achilles, Hercules, Romulus and Remus, etc.). In each case his origin is miraculous, conception takes place by non-human beings and birth is unnatural. The child is abandoned, becomes an orphan exposed to danger and may be mauled by animals. The child's activities are superhuman, he is invincible and hermaphroditic. All these characteristics can be found in Alan's material: the omnipotence with which he adhered to the theory—not mentioned so far—that it was God who created children and not mother and father; the god-baby who possessed miraculous powers—mainly destructive—featured in the baby's urine; next, there was a rupture of his relation to his mother, by whom he felt abandoned (cf. first interview supra). From very early on he lived in a dangerous world peopled by a big dangerous father and a bad witch-mother, and in his play there were monsters and devils, as well as God, who was liable to turn bad. The feeling of abandonment was further emphasized indirectly in his pre-occupation with orphans, openly expressed to his mother; it started with his asserting that another child who came to the clinic was an orphan and continued in the form of questions, which went on for some weeks. Invincibility was a characteristic of Alan's omnipotence and threats to it were reacted to with violence; furthermore, the fascination that he constellated all round him made possible unusual behaviour on his part that would not have been tolerated from others. Finally, there was the bisexuality of God, who could be either male or female.

The vulnerability of the hero—in myths he is depotentiated by something relatively insignificant—is related by Jung to the theme of 'smaller than the small yet greater than the great' and to the impotence of the child, which is compensated by his miraculous deeds.

Alan's vulnerability does not come out clearly in his interviews, but it would not be going too far to say that this was because it was so well compensated that I did not do anything to undermine it. It is true that he tended to react violently to disapproval (the first clinic interview showed this) and over soiling his pants or being physically punished he could be very upset and miserable; again, personal failure at school was scarcely bearable.

Jung's interpretation of the motif is as follows. He starts by pointing to the retrospective content of the child symbol: through it present experience is linked with the past. He defines the association in three ways: 1. As representing a memory of one's own childhood; 2. As a picture of certain forgotten things in childhood; 3. As the preconscious, childhood aspect of the collective psyche and 4. In a footnote he emphasizes the essentially irrational symbolic nature of the motif. Because he is analysing his material in terms of the archetype theory, he considers the third definition the best; in as much as he was working over organized myths from which personal elements have been removed he is correct; in doing so he had support from Kerényi who, in the same volume, ('The psychology of the child archetype' was published along with Kerényi's essay) argues that the myths refer to origins. But when myth-like material is produced by a patient, the separation of personal memories from impersonal collective determinants can only rarely be made; so, though Alan's myth-making sometimes looked like pure archetypal imagery, yet there were clear links with remembered incidents and to this must be added experience not remembered, for even if the links were not made explicitly by him they could easily be inferred. Therefore in this case, and indeed usually, the three definitions all apply, since all elements are closely interwoven (cf. Williams 1964).

Under another heading, Jung considers the 'potential future' inherent in the symbolic expressions and in this part he considers the child as a self symbol. It is archetypal in that it compensates the conscious attitude, especially when there is need to reunite conscious systems with their instinctual roots—a need that was evident and largely achieved in the development of Alan's case.

Inasmuch as Jung is referring to the material produced by adult patients, it is of interest that the same principles apply to Alan as well, for a child of his age has already developed all the essential structures that are characteristic of an adult.

But the child archetype not only compensates the ego in this way, it also foreshadows individuation. In the section on the futurity of the child archetype, Jung refers to the fact that self symbols can be observed in children's dreams; he uses them to support his idea that the 'synthesis' of the self is not an altogether suitable term and 'entelechy' is better to express the idea that there is an '*a priori* existence of potential wholeness'. I mention this because his idea is like my own formulation of primary self, differing from it, however, in that I would conceive the 'a priori' wholeness as the actual state of an infant. The difference may be accounted for in that Jung refers to the drive for unity that his adult cases revealed; he did not envisage clearly that this derived from the earliest state of a human being.

An interesting clinical conclusion can be drawn from these reflections. The individuating processes already in motion, as truly revealed in Alan's material, would account for the good result. It suggests that by the time Alan arrived for his treatment he was beginning to get well and under favourable circumstances this would have taken place anyway. There were already two favourable conditions in existence: the fortunate school environment and parents who were prepared to stand by him and get all the help they could.

It is not my intention to assert that the part taken by the analytic therapy was negligible, for it is clear there were specific instances when interpretations were mutative. Also the dialectic, which was never broken for long, was undoubtedly helpful to Alan, likewise the holding effect of the treatment-situation that regularly and reliably provided a place in which he could work out his main anxieties through behaviour that could not be tolerated at home. In spite of all this, reviewing the nature of Alan's material and its symbolism does suggest that all these were in a sense subsidiary: I did not cure the child but rather helped to provide conditions under which his own therapy was facilitated.

Reflection on archetypal processes does not complete what went on, for the activity of Alan's ego-functions was probably more significant in implementing his potential for health: his efforts to control his environment, often violently, and then his capacity to use pathways through which to establish relations, narcissistic and realistic, with his parents and myself; his use of the deintegrative processes in the self to make creative associations or to split off dangerous parts and set one against the other, combining with the most powerful ones against less threatening forms or enjoying the exercise of omnipotent power and the violence that this could generate. All this was progressively brought into relation with passive or actively loving feelings and impulses so that splitting defences became less necessary, and where it still took place it was channelled into socially and personally acceptable and more rewarding forms of living.

It may seem surprising that out of the material of a child who is so pathological the seeds of a healthy process can be discerned by studying the symbolism alone. In Alan's other material there was evidence of seriously defective maturation, of arrest at a stage in which omnipotence predominated, where objects were scarcely and sometimes not at all related to reality but to imaginative representation of his own needs. His mind was used more to sustain this state than to further fruitful, enjoyable and real achievement. The distinction between reality and his inner world was not developed and consequently, as we should say—as persons who had achieved this distinction, confused. There was inability to make use of frustration and often incapacity to tolerate it. He showed much evidence of reaction formation, of exhibitionistic defences, of repression and so on, and indeed the very extensive use of his imagination concealed the sources of pain and the traumatic experiences that lay behind it. Thus there had developed over his basic trauma, whose nature will be discussed later when his history is gone into, complex ego-structures from varying levels or stages of maturation right up to the oedipal. The use of analogies can and, I contend, has, in this case, cut through the complexities to the essential individuating processes relying on the self whose nature can be seen through it all.

Of course the deintegrating processes and the deintegrated parts had been used by Alan's ego to employ splitting defences, but these were a cloak and concealed the maturing drive that the self initiated under the influence of the environment.

It is relevant to note here that, apart from these theoretical reflections, it has for a long time been recognized that the delusions and hallucinations of adult schizophrenic cases show evidence of archetypal activity, and consequently they can be thought of as attempts at healing—a recent impressive study by Perry develops Jung's thesis. The part of symbol formation in infant development has likewise long been known and was graphically stated by Klein in a short paper (1930). It was developed by Segal (1957). The importance of recognizing this can scarcely be overstressed in a case like Alan. How he developed is in part related in the case-description and some further indication of it is given in the follow-up communication (cf. p. 242f infra).

Body-Mind and Infantile Sexuality

Alan's mother once remarked that her son did not seem aware of his body, he would never say if he was thirsty, and he did not seem to notice if he was cold. This observation crystallized a number of impressions I had been grouping together. I had noticed that he did not complain when he was hurt by banging against an object in the room; an object he fell back on to and then slithered down onto the floor. The event was quite alarming and his mother leaped up with a warm exclamation, wanting to come to his aid. He must have been quite badly bruised but he jumped up, ignored his mother and came into the play-room as if nothing had happened. Nor did he show any signs of distress during the interview: he played, rather more quietly than usual, at a theme he had been developing, that of world destruction, but it did not show unusual characteristics.

Another striking event was the following. One day, when coming to the clinic, Alan jumped off the bus while it was still going and fell flat on the pavement, bruising himself quite badly (especially his head); again, he must have hurt himself severely. Again, he treated it as if it had never happened, and it took a lot of work to get him to express his fury with the bus conductor. Only next day did he complain of a pain in his head.

The way in which he used his mind and his fantasy to control pain was characteristic, and the incident with the bus illustrates it. As he arrived at the top of the stairs at the clinic, he said to the secretary: 'That was a dangerous thing to do, jumping off that bus.' He came into my room rather shocked and pale, and sat in the chair for a bit before going over to the sand-tray. I knew nothing, beyond what he had said, at this juncture. The water-play then began in a familiar way: first ordinary sea, then magic sea, which was much more personified than usual; it could be talked to and controlled, it got angry and raged—the waves became big, but he would say 'Be calm, sea', and then the waves would go down. Finally, the sea became Minnek.

A story ran through his play starting 'a long, long time ago.' At first the sea endangered lots of people, but soon there was only one person—a soldier, who at first liked swimming very much and the sea was wonderful, *but it became dangerous later and he* 'jumped off' into it. Thus the soldier was probably Alan, as it was he who jumped off the bus. In the end, when the sea was Minnek, *the soldier got into the bucket but Minnek washed him out of it. At the end he concluded 'and he came in the end to Quisley.'* (The italicized passages are additions to a usual theme.) He then told me that I am 'there to look after him'.

On the basis that he felt I was safe, I translated that he was expressing his feelings about coming by bus to the clinic. Response: 'I don't like that bus conductor and never shall. I wish he were drowned in Minnek.' Then he went on to detail the depth and bottomlessness of the sea; later, chewing Plasticine, he concluded that the conductor 'is a great bad magician; he turns the boy into a monster and he eats up the other one'.

All this suggested to me that his body-image was at times, if not always, defective, either because of denial or alternatively because it had not developed well.

According to the theory of the self that I was working on, deintegration leads to the formation of ego-nuclei round the oral, anal and genital zones especially. In the course of maturation they become linked to form a body-image by a complex of processes. Though anatomically the zones are separated and serve distinct and different functions, this is *not* how a baby experiences them; the knowledge has to be acquired. At first, it may be assumed experiences are registered in terms of pleasure and pain, very little located in space or time, and so similar experiences are treated as identical. Because of this, states of excitement in the zones are very much mixed up with each other; this was reflected in Alan's play-activities and in the fantasies that went with them. The distinguishing of different kinds of excitement no doubt grows by repeated experience but they cannot be completely located and differentiated until a body-image is formed; this involves perception and cathexis of the skin-surface. A number of circumstances contribute to this, of which a most important one is provision by the mother of physical holding, especially in periods of instinctual excitement but also during less excited states, and so affectionate physical interchanges between her and her infant, such as cuddling. In Alan's case it is likely that this was disturbed (cf. infra p. 242).

Another idea that occurred to me derived from his seeming lack of feeling about the inside of his body. It is reasonable to think that until the body-image is formed there can be no experience of an inner world in a body sense. Since this body-image is assumed to exist before an inner world of imagination and thought and feeling, it will be readily understood that in these spheres there can be as yet no sense of their inner nature. If infant experiences cannot be located but are rather experienced as pleasure and pain, similarity and difference, there would be a basis for representation of experience in terms of the symbolic equations so frequent in Alan's play. They were nearly all objective in the sense that there was no reference to him and, if there was as yet no stable body-image sufficiently organized, the objects in his play could not be referred to him either. Following up this idea it would seem that, though anatomically the zones are separate from each other (and this is discovered through the differing kinds of excitement and environmental response), yet they are also very much mixed up in feeling and so in play; this meant, in Alan's case, that representations of them were located in his mind.

Alan's impulsivness can also be made sense of in the light of the idea that his body-image was defective. He acted on the basis of an affect linked to an idea or image and there was little resistance because he could not contain it; there was nowhere to put it inside, and so he tended to hit out, throw an object, pull hair, etc., without restraint. I do not, of course, mean that this was always so but it was a state of affairs that predominated. But let us return to the idea that Alan's activities were mainly controlled by his mind. The relation between his body-feeling, his impulses and his imagination is not easy to describe. When he was playing, his main creative mental and physical activity, his actions were closely linked with the imagery he was developing. So long as he felt I was understanding him and so, one might say, going along with him in his mind, his often considerable excitement was mostly manageable. So there became established a field of activity and imagination going on between us, which was safe enough because I was there, as he once put it, 'to look after him.'

In these activities there were indications of anxieties whose intensity could only be hinted at and amongst them the libidinal zones were clearly important: they can now be considered.

Genital Zone

There was much fantasy about babies' urine, rain, floods, etc., which might suggest urethral excitement, but very little took place and in interviews he seldom wanted to urinate; at home he had not complete control over his urine. Separation between his body and fantasy is to be seen in his statements: it was never he who made the dangerous floods or fertilized the desert, it was always God or the babies. In this first part of his treatment, however, some events indicated that the dissociation was not complete. Thus from time to time he would hold his penis, as if to stop either the discharge of urine or an erection. Once he poured rather a lot of water on the floor; I stopped him, he at once held his penis and then there developed the following story-game:

'And there was a monster', he announced and he took some Plasticine off the wall, where he had previously stuck it, and swished it about in the water. When it broke in two, he exclaimed, 'Oh, the monster is broke'. The monster, however, remained sufficiently viable to eat a fish, but was again injured, so it went to hospital. It was operated on, was cut into bits and 'that's the end of the monster'.

Within the complexity of this fantasy was a clear indication of a feeling in his penis when I stopped him flooding the floor. What kind of feeling? The story suggests castration-anxiety, linked to oral systems and possibly anal ones as well (his use of Plasticine to indicate a monster). The fantasy suggests that castration-anxieties followed genital activity, though in a generalized way we could say he was a 'phallic' personality.

The mental linking together of zones, i.e. sources of excitement, is characteristic of a deintegrate because it is conceived as part of the whole (the self). In early stages of development, the separation and conscious placing of organs within the body-image does not exist but the deintegrative discharge does focus a priority in one zone. Thus in this bit of play the focus was on Alan's penis but anal and oral feelings were referred to or included. His sexual anxieties were suggested also by his reaction to interpretation of the primal scene, which subsequent events confirmed (cf. p. 232 infra). Taken in the aggregate these reflections indicate that Alan's genital organization was not well established.

Anal Zone

Before he came to the clinic, and during a large part of his treatment, he was faecally incontinent about once a week. At home, but not at the clinic, he spent long periods in the lavatory where he used large quantities of paper, though how he used it can only be surmised, as he would allow nobody into the lavatory. Mother also reported that if he marked his pants he would insist on their being changed at once.

In this first part of therapy his fantasies of dangerous, poisonous faeces, ejected by the baby-god, were a main feature of his compulsive manic action with sand and Plasticine. His most hectically violent struggles were with the magic witch-mother; if in his excitement he filled up the sink with sand so that the waste pipe was blocked, he attributed the blocking to her; the struggle was then intensified till she was overcome and done away with.

Besides this aggressive significance of faeces, there was another feeling about them that gradually came to the fore. It was related to their softness: he would stroke and mould the sand-faeces that would then become 'the soft mummy's breast'. The equation between 'mother's' faeces and food led to tasting games in which he expressed and developed his feelings of disgust and revulsion for sand or Plasticine; the positive relation between the two led to his developing games centring on the poem 'Baker's man'.

From all this is can be seen that the anal impulses that gave rise to his incontinence were mainly symbolized. In this first part of his therapy he never defaecated during the interviews, nor did he become anally excited during his games; it was only at home that he occasionally soiled his pants. It therefore seems that there were anxieties that were dealt with by fantasy-elaboration and denial—it is not me but the god-baby. As in the genital zone, there was thus evidence that the maturation of anal organization was arrested.

Oral Organization

By contrast there was much to suggest that his oral organization had gone forward quite well. He was rather easy about his mouth, and mine too, in the first interview; he could use his mouth for eating and tasting toffee-sand by chewing Plasticine in the interview. He would spit water and he could slobber; he would stroke his tongue and he would say if his mouth felt 'horrid inside'. Soon after his treatment began, he became easy about his mother's breasts, talking to her about them with pleasure and wanting to stroke them. But he was not entirely without oral anxieties for, right at the start, when he was looking inside boxes he thought there was something inside them that might bite. Later he started biting toys as part of the working through of this anxiety and once put a toy in my mouth, expressing surprise that I did not bite it.

Muscle and Skin Erotism

There remains the very active use of his muscles, which must have conveyed a sense of himself as legs and arms, but this would not have been maintained during less active states. Once he came and sat in my lap in the first interview; he did not come to be cuddled but to examine and attack a localized part of me: my face. One could say that in this part of me and himself there was a sense of a bit of body-image developing, though it had not extended beyond his face: he put his cheek against mine, deriving pleasure from so doing, so there was a sense of having a surface; and he looked inside my mouth and so experienced my having an inside. This was followed up by looking in other objects: these were related to teeth, for he said, 'It might bite'.

Discussion

Alan did not draw people; indeed, he drew very little, and then what he produced was maps. If he had drawn a self-portrait, it might have been of a face, with emphasized mouth and nose, leg and arms; in short, like the pictures small children draw before a trunk is added. The unorganized state of Alan's body-image and the failure of maturation to take place in the anal and genital drives are important for understanding the nature of Alan's condition. His rather good and ambivalent relation to his mother as breast suggests that there had been a good start to his life as a baby and that the trauma, whatever it was, had taken place later, possibly when the splints were applied to his feet; mother thought she had been too rough, but, if true, there was surprisingly little reference to all this in his material. Moreover, Alan said that he remembered what she did to him, so it may have been conscious. Whether this was important or not, a great deal more must have contributed. But the excessive use of projective identification ('living in a mad world'), his ruthlessness and absence of concern, pining or depression, combined with the fragmentation of his body-image, all suggest that the damage took place before the second year. The integrity of the body-image is closely related to self-feeling, to the sense of identity: Alan's violence, his omnipotence, as well as the projective identification, could all be partly understood on the basis that his self-feeling was exceedingly precarious. But if this was so, how can the presence of self-imagery be understood?

In my view, it requires the assumption of a primary unity, a given state from which the infant begins, before the ego has become established. It is this unity of the self that leads to early object-relations being all parts of the self (deintegrates). At first there is no external object, nor for that matter any internal ones, only a state of primary identity between self and the infant's environment. It is from this that infantile omnipotence derives and also his violence, for anything that is not-self is treated as alien and to be destroyed. It is only through maturation and good mothering that the infant gradually recognizes the difference between self and not-self and the primary self converted into symbolic representations. This had taken place in Alan but the representations were mental— it was as if the unity of the self were perpetuated in his mind, which treated objects as self or not-self. If they did not fit his omnipotent self-feeling, they were treated as alien—hence the predominance of violence in an attempt to destroy or triumph over them.

The fact of symbolization in imagery, verbal or visual, means that there is consciousness and so it is necessary also to recognize ego-functions, which were quite considerable in Alan's case, particularly his capacity for thought. They were, however, linked up and influenced all along by affects and close to the self. The unity was represented in finding sameness in difference; the deintegrative function of the self was being used by the ego to further its splitting and fragmentating defences.

The particular splittings that Alan exhibited were manic: rapid and excited shifts or struggles, with ever-increasing violence to overcome a bad object, which was separate and different from a good one. The pattern again suggests early traumata, for the depressive position has not been reached, or, if it has, it is being violently defended against; it is too dangerous to recognize an object as having good and bad characteristics—these must be kept separate. It seems possible, therefore, that Alan was defending himself against a feeling of hopelessness and despair.

Acting Out

Acting out was a prominent feature all along. Because of his impulsiveness, my objective was to avoid stopping any activity but this became impossible in one period of the treatment.

As his play became more and more excited, his fear of retaliation and punishment by me came into the open. I interpreted that he was comparing my room and myself with his home and his parents and that he expected me to punish him as they did. I developed this theme in detail and, as his fear of punishment became less, concurrently his omnipotent fantasies became more open and difficult to control. I have already said how he filled the sand-tray with water, making the biggest sea in the world, called 'Minnek'. Storms were announced and waves were made by rocking the tray back and forth. These activities became increasingly violent, so that water would splash over onto the floor. I interpreted that he feared his good doctor-father (myself) would not survive and that I would turn into the totally bad, angry, dangerous father that he knew at home. As the interpretations began to allay his anxiety, he tested me by throwing more and more water on the floor or at me personally. I tried to deal with the situation by mopping up the water but he would swish over more than could be coped with; it seeped under the door of the play-room and finally ran through the floor into the room below, provoking protests from the staff working there. A confrontation was inevitable: I explained why the floods must stop and employed a number of manoeuvres like turning off the tap or the stop-cock or the pipe to the tap. He was not to be outdone and he angrily responded in kind, till I eventually became angry and shook him. He went passive, frightened and bewildered and it took him a considerable time to recover.

When the immediate shock had passed, I began making interpretations about how he compared me with his father and I said his terror was due to my becoming much more like him than he had expected. In later interviews I kept on referring to the event, until he asked what it was that made me angry. I answered the question and also told him that he could ask because he was beginning to suspect that my anger was reliable, because it had not happened again, and that he wanted to know whether I thought so too. A short time later he took issue with his own father about being punished and after this he was treated differently. It therefore seems that the trauma had been healed as a result of my method of treating him.

After this episode, the flooding stopped for a short time, but he soon started again, recognizing that he could not control his excitement; I arranged with him that when it began I would take the sand-tray out of the room and in this he came to collaborate.

In arranging a treatment-room, the problem is to make it represent something like home but yet be sufficiently different to keep it clear that this *is* a treatment-room and so different from home.

The problem Alan confronted me with was whether the room could have been altered so as not to make a treatment atmosphere that was provocative. There is nothing desirable about mess and violence in themselves, but they are sometimes necessary in order to understand what it is all about and so that the conflicts over such behaviour can be resolved. Therefore they do not need encouragement. If there are pleasant and comfortable chairs, tables and a couch that can be spoiled, this is enough to indicate that the analyst cares about what happens to the room, but the furniture must be strong enough to stand being jumped on or even turned over.

The painted walls and ceiling made them easy to clean rapidly so that each time he came it started by looking clean and pleasant, showing that I cared, like his parents, about the room being agreeable for him.

A major problem was the amount of water. The room could have been made waterproof without spoiling it and an inconspicuous drain could have been put in to prevent excessive accumulation of fluid. But, in addition, the floor near the door would need to have been raised to prevent water flowing underneath it.

The treatment room was, however, to be used by other children and, however rapidly it could be cleaned up, signs of mess, such as a wet floor, could not have been avoided. For this reason, for much of the time I arranged for Alan to be the last patient.

But what alterations could have been made? First of all, the overflow from the sink could have been sufficiently large to drain off water as fast as the tap discharged water into it. As the overflow is usually of standard size, it would be better to have the inflow restricted, to prevent the sink being filled up so that it overflows.

Finally, there was a rather large sand-tray on legs. It could be wheeled about and rocked. This had to be removed and Alan was not in the end averse from this. Why have it there at all?

There are therapists who lay great stress on it; among Jungians Kalff, in particular, uses it extensively, in combination with a large collection of toys. The child selects what he wants to use and as a result constructs symbolic patterns, often of considerable interest and therapeutic value. For this reason, and also because small children enjoy it, there is good reason for having a tray available, but I do not think it helped much in Alan's case. It was his anal and urethral anxieties, and the violence connected with them, that were important, not the sand and water in themselves; in addition Alan did not take pleasure in constructive achievement, except in making stories, which sand, water and toys illustrated.

There was one other feature in the technique I was using at the time that Alan forced me to change. The toys were kept in a cupboard and were used by other children. Alan never cared about them and was frequently destructive with them because they were shared. Subsequently I changed this and never had a pool of toys but a separate cupboard for each child, so that he could treat them as his own and could add to them or discard them as he wished. Later on (cf. p. 230 infra) it became very clear how important it was to Alan that I saw other children and it seems clear that the common pool of toys was a forcible reminder that he dared not put into words.

These reflections apply particularly to children like Alan in whom splitting processes are a particular feature; in children whose self-image is more organized the problem is not so acute but it is there all the same, even though it is not acted out because conflicts are contained and can be more easily understood.

Improvements

During this part of Alan's treatment there were changes that his parents and schoolteacher reported. The most relevant ones were in relation to his mother: soon after the interviews began there was a marked improvement in their relationship; the barrier she felt so distressing almost disappeared, and Alan became increasingly affectionate, and when there was a quarrel it was less intense. He became interested in her body and especially her breasts, which he stroked; and instead of only abusing her he would say: 'I love my mother very much so I must do everything she tells me' or 'Lovely mummy . . . mummy . . .'. Sometimes he would talk baby-talk to her, using words she used to the new baby, and the relationship with his brothers became less violent and sometimes affectionate. There seemed little doubt that the change came first from Alan but at the same time his mother, encouraged by his affectionate approaches, became less depressed and responded to her son's love; in addition, her overall resentment, anger and hostility towards him altered, to become more closely related to specific incidents: it became short-lived instead of continuous. There was also a movement forward by Alan into more direct oedipal patterns, especially at home—hatred of his father and love for his mother appeared. This had not been mentioned before; on the contrary,

Alan's mother had reported that he turned to his father and away from her.

How does this relate to Alan's therapy? Right from the start (first interview), his suspicion of and lack of trust in his mother came into the open, and later his violent attack on the witch-mother seemed to be the most significant theme relevant to Alan's relation to her. The division (splitting) of parents into good and bad and the overtly pregenital ruthless relation to his real mother make it clear that the conflicts had been mainly pre-oedipal.

The treatment had first contained these early conflicts and then worked on them sufficiently to release his sensual enjoyment of his mother; most of all it was a part of her (breast); there his pleasure became generalized into love. Concurrently ongoing individuating processes based on the self led into oedipal patterns most evident at home but also in the interviews.

SECTION THREE

It was my refusal to allow so much acting out that partly led to more controlled activities, so that he would play in the sand and use water in a much more moderate fashion. Making up stories became a central feature of the interview and when the end of it was announced by me he would impersonate a radio announcer and close down the performance. He had adopted a way of organizing his thoughts and fantasies that was familiar to him: for some time he had been writing stories at home. His mother once offered to bring them, but never did so; these stories, she said, contained 'private words'.

The stories he made up in his interviews were various and he illustrated them with suitable activities. They would begin with an introduction such as 'A long time ago . . .' or 'Oh there was a monster . . .' and there was one about a couple 'Rowing down the river on a Sunday afternoon'. All these stories started during the manic defence period but became much more ritualized later. 'Rowing down the river on a Sunday afternoon' usually started blissfully but then there would be some threat or a disaster: 'There is a boat with two people in it and they have oars; they sing "Rowing down the river on the Sunday afternoon . . ." A storm starts'. Then he rocked the sand-tray, remarking 'Look out—a big wave!' and 'It's God making the storm;' then the waves got bigger. . . . Will the boat sink? It did and the couple were thrown into the water.

Another story started from a desert: 'The sand is a desert; it becomes the world. Countries are in it: Greece and Troy, with England a long way away—10,000 miles'. Plasticine was cut up and the bits represented the countries of the world. In the end Minnek was created, the countries were scooped out and thrown into it.

A longer one developed as follows: he came in chewing something, which he threw out of the window. 'The desert is not very safe—C (a person) can eat lorries. This is where C lives among the trees; he has gone for a walk in the desert; he went somewhere to hide in the sand, but when a criminal comes along he might come back.' Alan then started eating Plasticine and became very excited. 'Which part of the desert is he in? I don't know. I'm going to have lunch, I want some people to eat; yum, yum, delicious. That's C's lunch—very dangerous; he'll eat you and bite you to death. I've had enough.' After a pause another theme began; in it a 'lovely flood' started, which washed his home away.

There were still violent outbursts; bombing attacks on cities, men getting killed, but these were all controlled, as it were, by the story and there was never the same flooding and the mess was very much reduced. Indeed, a time came when he began to help regularly in clearing up the now rather small amounts of sand and water on the floor.

In this period there were some developments that worked into the fourth part of his treatment. He started to ask for physical contact. It began when, interrupting some aggressive play, he announced one day that he was 'coming to talk' to me; he ran over to where I was sitting and lay across me, wriggling about with pleasure. He subsequently became interested in my pipe and its smoke, which he disliked because, he said, it made him cough. He also made statements like 'You are here to look after me' or 'I love you'.

There then developed games of being chased and caught and from time to time he wanted me to pick him up in my arms like a baby, turn him upside down and lower him down onto the floor, which he likened to being born. At this time there was more phallic play: men started to shoot each other and animals.

Jealousy and Possessiveness

During this period Alan became more and more possessive and jealous. He was angry if I was not ready to see him directly he arrived and he would bang on the door or even burst into the room. Interpreting the reasons for this led to modification of his behaviour; his activities became diverted to the end of the interview when he would turn the tables and chairs upside down*. I interpreted that he was determined that I should not see any other children—he was to be the only one; but, further than this, the room represented the inside of his mother, the horrible mother who twice before had had babies inside when he was little and who might have them again. There were a number of indications of this in his play: there had been violent maltreatment of dolls and the theme had run through his earlier fantasies of the witch-mother. I related all this to him as follows: he suspected that I had children of my own and might turn into a horrible mother and have other babies (the other children that he knew came to my room raised these thoughts). I further told him that this was how he had felt when his mother carried babies inside her and that if he suspected she was going to have another one he would again feel like destroying the baby and everything else inside her. The pain he remembered at his brother's birth, when he was small, was too horrible and he could not bear it to happen again.

This long and complex interpretation was possible because he went along with it and kept adding to and amplifying my communications so that what was initiated by me became a combined effort to understand how he felt. As he worked through his fears he began to regress, demanding to be carried out of the room in my arms. He would curl up in them, calling himself my 'baby' and sucking away with his mouth, putting either his thumb or some other object into it.

Faecal Incontinence

Before this play developed he would often start putting his hand over his anus and at the same time he held his penis. A

---

* This was taking up a bit of play that he had started early on in his treatment: he would turn the chairs and tables over, put all the toys away in the cupboard and then sit in front of it. I had not understood it at the time but in the present context its meaning was very clear.

dreamy look came into his eyes and eventually instead of playing with me he passed faeces of varying consistency. One lot made a soft mass on the floor. This was difficult to manage because it seemed to be a present, but it was so repulsive that I could not conceal my revulsion. I had said that he was wanting to give me a present of ah-ahs (faeces) and he became decidedly ironic about it: when he passed the soft mass he said: 'Present for Dr. Fordham!', giving me the impression that he meant something like 'If you think that is a present, what are you going to do about it?'. So I told him it might be a present but it smelt and was better put in the lavatory: when a dreamy look came on I took him to the lavatory and there followed rather long sessions, using quantities of lavatory paper, as his mother had reported. It was after this episode had been negotiated that he showed more and more evidence of homosexual impulses and I eventually began to interpret them as an aspect of the primal scene.

A bit of behaviour by Alan's mother at this time was rather striking. Before his faecal incontinence at the clinic she had commented on his improvement, but she never made reference to Alan's state when he came home after his clinic session. Large quantities of faeces had been passed by Alan and they were sometimes bulky and soft; they must have made his pants filthy. Why did she never say anything, for it would have been useful if she had brought clean pants for him to change into? This very suggestive behaviour clearly meant a very close relation between her and Alan over his incontinence; perhaps she thought I knew nothing about it and she was being a loyal mother by keeping his supposed secret.

SECTION FOUR

One day Alan asked me to come to the sand-tray and showed me a woman in the sand; the little lumps were her soft breasts. Then there was a woman under the water, drowned. Her husband was there; he was 'a good swimmer, a man of the sea'. He did not like his wife. I reflected, without saying anything, that he may not have liked her soft faecal breasts.

There then followed much aggressive play between two people and one was kicked away. He started pouring water into the sand and onto the floor, and then dug about more in the sand, which he called 'making bogs'; at the same time he passed faeces, which dropped down his trousers onto the floor so that there was a mixture of sand and faeces. At this time he became altogether more friendly.

I interpreted that, in the fights between men, one getting kicked away (there was quite a lot of kicking at this period) meant there was denial of their wanting to mix their 'bogs' together. I said that when he had told me 'I will never love my father', it was because he felt his father (and I too) wanted to do this with him; he also wanted to join in a fearful mixing of bogs, but dared not. He showed me this by making his own bogs with his behind and digging out sand ('my bogs') with his hand and throwing it on the floor so that the two mixed together.

After throwing sand on the floor and defaecating, he went back to the fights between men, but this time the sheriff and the police featured. The game petered out when I interpreted the relation between the two, i.e. that he had become anxious (afraid) of what I was talking about and wanted it stopped (hence the introduction of the sheriff and the police).

This play indicated that the aggressive conflict related to the things two people do or do not do together with parts of their bodies; breasts and faeces entered into it.

Twice before, this subject had been broached: the first time was early on in Part I. Alan built in the sand a round house with a door, a window and a chimney. Then two people fought in front of it and one pushed himself into the house near the front door. I interpreted that the one going in was daddy's jimmy pushing into mother to make babies. This statement was meaningful to him for he stopped the object pushing in and destroyed the house. I was surprised at the violence and said no more because of the amount of aggression that was mobilized. In the light of later developments of primal-scene fantasies this interpretation must have been both incomplete and inaccurate; it had not touched on the complexities of his feeling, which only appeared in this fourth part. It is likely that the most significant part of what I said was the mention of babies, for the idea of intercourse was at that early time remote from his consciousness.

About six months after this, a game developed of putting a

bus in the water. Two people would be put on top of it and they would be washed off. One day there was a change in the play and he put an engine in the water and pushed it backwards and forwards. I interpreted this as his wish to have daddy's jimmy and push it backwards and forwards in mummy as he had been 'told' daddy did to make a baby. He did not dissent this time but for the first time he ended the interview early. It appeared that my use of the word 'told' had been more on the mark than I could have known, for the day before his parents had actually given him detailed sexual information. He appeared not to take it in for, when they enquired so as to be sure he had understood, he said he had 'forgotten' and reverted to his own ideas that God sent babies.

About one month before this there had been some play that suggested primal-scene fantasies from a different level. One day he was being incontinent and had himself talked about soft sand being like anal feelings; he made a soft hill in his play. A pole was put up on it and an animal came; first it sank into the sand and then ploughed through the hill. I interpreted this as his parents being together in some way but this did not alter the play, which went on much the same till, in the end, the whole hill was ploughed into and messed up. There followed floods and a tide that threatened to swamp the hill, but they receded; the hill then became a rock and the pole was restored. My interpretation of this had been that he knew about the messes that mothers and babies made together and perhaps he felt mummy and daddy did something like it, especially through daddy pushing into her, as he could imagine I did with Mrs. Fordham. In contrast to the earlier occasions, he agreed to what I said and his play became more active.

It therefore seemed that his defences had become less strong as his anal associations, feelings and fantasies became more acceptable—less revolting and disgusting. This idea had, I thought, been part of his messy acting out, which had now ceased altogether.

Some time after this he said his bombs were magic but 'they don't kill'. He had a stick of bombs in his anus but also number two is a present. Interpretation: so the bombs are jimmy bombs. In reply he shouted 'Yes, that's right', and later: 'I do not give him (daddy) my jimmy'. He played in the soft sand. By this time the soft sand was known to represent the soft feelings in his anus—the idea had been agreed between us. Interpretation: 'The soft sand is the soft feeling in your bottom when it wants my jimmy to push in'; this was with reference to some play in which he was pushing a man into the sand and killing others. Interpretation: 'So daddy is bad (the man that got killed) because he gives mummy his jimmy and not you'. Then one day he was making a soft place in the sand and became very seductive, dreamy and looking anxiously and appealingly at me, so I made the following interpretation. 'Your bottom sometimes feels that it wants daddy's jimmy in it, just as you sometimes like now, want mine also. But you fear that if it got inside it would turn bad and damage you, like the bogs, which were like several jimmies that you push onto the floor.'

This led on to talking about his wish to be a mother and at this time he announced that he had a breast in his shoulder and he bared it, wanting, indeed urging me, to suck and enjoy it; it pleased him when I pretended to do so.

At this time he was becoming even more friendly, showing that his anxieties about me had lessened; so when he again, with more zest and less anxiety, played with the soft sand, pushing an object into it, I interpreted that daddy's jimmy had now become good, and mine too, and that he would like to have my jimmy in his bottom and enjoy it as mummy did too. He responded first with close attention to what I was saying and then with delight; he lay on his back on the floor with his legs apart, like a woman inviting intercourse, at the same time asking me to 'say that again about the jimmy'.

I interpreted that my words represented to him my good jimmy and that they made good feelings in his anus that he wanted to feel again and again. The interview ended happily.

The last interpretation depended on my feeling, backed up by theory but I did not have one overtly in my mind at the time for it seemed evident that it was my words that produced the effect on his body, as indeed he recognized by his reply: 'Say that again.' I do not think, however, that I could have followed his acts so carefully if I had not in the back of my mind had the idea that an archetype is bipolar: at one pole there are physical impulses (his acts) and at the other representations of them—the words.

At about the time of these developments in Alan's analysis, his mother recorded improvements at home. She remarked that

Alan's incontinence had stopped altogether. After working over his homosexuality, which was now seen and understood as identification with his mother in intercourse, his attitude to his father changed and, though he still got angry with him, it did not last and he soon became friendly again.

SECTION FIVE

The activities at this stage were clearly sadistic and worked through in angry jealousy and envy of his parents' sexual activities and the body-parts they used in them. During it he was so absorbed that he said practically nothing. First, there were two animals that fought each other and this was interpreted as animal parents that represented his own parents. Next he took a screwdriver, heated it in the fire and attacked a male bull, who was very fierce, and a female cow; he attacked the udders of the cow and the genital region of the bull. But he also attacked the cow's shoulder (which he had previously connected with the breast), legs and thigh, all of which had holes burnt in them. The bull was the active one; he attacked other animals but first was warded off and then they were killed. The reason for all this ferocity only became explicit once, when the game introduced humans: there was a man who put 'poison' into the 'mother cow', and then the usual violence followed.

When I interpreted this play as anger at his parents combined to exclude him, a calf was added to it and he was spared from the attacking screwdriver as well as from attack by the bull. The next step was to introduce a war-dance and war-drums and the fighting couple were again violently attacked, by the warriors. The interpretation that ended this phase was as follows: 'You are glad to know about good brave fighters because one day you hope to be one. You sing and bang on the floor to make yourself strong enough to attack daddy's hot burning jimmy and drive it out. You can't always do it now because you partly want to join in and attack that bad dangerous hot mummy (the fire and mother-animals)'.

After this he took a male and a female toy animal under the table and, keeping his body between them and me, put them

235

together lovingly. I told him this loving of animal parents was possible because he was protecting them from me, into whom he had put all his bad wishes.

I could use this idea of putting bad wishes into me because he had introduced it early in the treatment and I had used it afterwards from time to time. It all began at home when t here was a conflict over going to bed. When taken there, he had said to his mother, 'I don't like you and I don't like daddy' and (half crying), 'I've got prickly feelings in my eyes'. His mother said that he mustn't go to bed feeling like that or he would have bad dreams, to which he replied, '*You'll* have the bad dreams; I'm going to give them to you', and he made magic movements with his hands. After this he liked mummy and went to sleep happily. A few days later he had talked to me about dreams, saying that he thought his parents or God put them into his thoughts.

It may seem surprising that this was the first time he mentioned the dreams, which he occasionally told to his mother. He once told his mother that he had had a dream in which he was with his younger brother, John, and that a volcano had erupted. He had taken hold of John's hand and run to safety. All the hills around were black and he did not touch them because if he did they would burn his hands. Mother suggested: 'Why don't you tell your dream to Dr. Fordham? I think he would be interested', but Alan thought differently: 'Oh no, it's much too strange to tell Dr. Fordham!' Mother said in reply that she did not think it was and that it was an interesting dream. Alan's interest in dreams was real enough, for it also appeared in a story he wrote later on for his school magazine. That he did not tell them to me was part of his transference-feeling. At that time he did not often tell them at all and it may be that, in the treatment, the affect that went into dreams at night went into his play and activities and that it was like Jung's observation that active imagination can replace dreams.

Confirmation of this view was given when working over his pregenital primal-scene fantasies, including the idea of urinary intercourse, which I had interpreted. It was then that he said: 'I have too many dreams at night, I dream of the sea!' He then spilt water on the floor, sucked some in, spat on a chair; next he played at the two people in a boat and made a storm till the boat was sunk.

SECTION SIX

After the primal-scene fantasies had been ended Alan's play started to centre on the conflict of opposites, between good and bad groups of people. He arranged fierce battles between cowboys and Indians in which the battles were often indecisive. Besides this play, he started writing out long stories, one of them being about a large band of thugs who made fires and explosions. Many police were killed but many thugs themselves were killed in their own explosions and in the buildings in a town they set on fire. Reinforcements of police arrived and eventually the robbers retired to their hideout, and there they were in danger. The fantasies were always lengthy and dramatic, but the 'baddies' were eventually, if not eliminated, at least repulsed or driven away.

SECTION SEVEN

The End of Therapy

For some time before treatment ended, Alan's parents had been feeling that they wanted and were able to take responsibility for their child. I had not committed myself, but when a summer holiday arrived I thought this might be a useful occasion to test Alan's capacity to adapt without me. On previous holidays Alan had become more difficult during the break in treatment, more violent and intractable; he would improve when his visits to the clinic started again. So, if the holiday went well, this favoured ending; if it did not, then further treatment was indicated.

During the holiday in question, Alan sent me a postcard saying what a good holiday he was having: he had been climbing mountains and was 'just off to collect cockles'. The postcard was, I thought, an expression of a continuing friendliness that had been developing in his analysis and that with me continuing in his mind he could enjoy himself without my being physically present.

His parents' report, when they returned to the clinic, agreed with what he wrote—it had been a good family holiday, the

best they had ever experienced. Alan was helpful and co-operative and, indeed, if there had been anybody to worry about,
it was their youngest son and not Alan. It was after hearing his
parent's report that I saw Alan again; I told him my thoughts
about his postcard and added that as he could be happy with
his family when I was not there, he might consider stopping
coming to see me.

There was no direct response. He started a game he had been
playing before his holiday—animals were threatened by men
or devils, who were smoke. Mysteriously, the animals kept
getting killed—eleven were reduced to four, and then he started
asking how much more time there was. I interpreted that he
wanted to be sure that I would control the devils if he could not.
Further that he also had felt that I was a devil attacking his
genitals and his anus when I told him about the idea of stopping.
This also made him feel, as he used to, that there were devils
in his jimmy and his number two. This interpretation was indicated because he had been holding his penis and fingering his
trousers over his anus in a way that had been worked over
between us earlier. His game continued; the animals were
reduced to one but this one conquered the devils, and brought
the dead animals to life. Alan asserted as this happened: 'So
the good powers overcame the evil'.

In the next interview the destruction was much less. I continued as usual: interpreting his pleasure that I had understood
his belief that he could control the devil (urine and faeces) and
his evil parents, and could want to be good and feel good himself,
and that I was no longer necessary to him. He looked pleased
and proud of himself, so I told him the next time would be the
last.

In this last interview, he was more friendly and open than
before, and there was even less destruction. The interview ended
as follows. When I announced the end he got behind a chair
and the excited look, which went with violently turning the
furniture over, came into his eyes. After an internal struggle,
he jumped on the table and the interview ended with my
carrying him out on my shoulders and down the passage to
his mother, with whom he went off down the stairs.

Mother and father came together for a final interview.
There was not much I could say. They had already been convinced Alan could be treated like their other children but they

asked me whether there was anything special I could suggest that would help him. To this I said in substance that I would suggest treating him as a normal member of their family and that special treatment was no longer indicated. It turned out to be important that I underlined their view but I left the door open for them to bring up any special situation that might arise.

The use of 'normal' did not, of course, apply in the conventional sense but rather to the family norm. So in talking to Alan's parents I was relying upon a number of features of the family life.

Alan's father, a statistician of high intelligence, and the paternal grandfather were both in many ways like Alan. They tended to cut themselves off from other people and to make arbitrary decisions relevant to the family. They both suffered from moods and bad temper. The grandfather, it was said, had recovered from a 'nervous breakdown' and there had been much hostility between him and Alan's father, who was consequently understanding of his son's aggression towards him.

This combination of characteristics made for a home environment that was not too 'normal' for Alan to live in and at the same time was basically healthy. Furthermore, significant changes had taken place in the parents during therapy. If they made attempts to push Alan to behave too well for his capacity and he showed distress signals, they had come to understand what was beyond his ability to achieve. In addition, Alan's mother had come to understand that often her intolerance of Alan was related to her own personal difficulties and that these were related to her own childhood and the way she had been brought up.

Post-Analytic Treatment

As it turned out, not unexpectedly, after several months Alan's parents contacted the clinic about the situation at school. To understand why this was necessary, a review of the situation there will help.

When Alan first went to the school at the age of five, he sat at the back of the class and seemed to pay little attention. Soon, however, his talented and perceptive classmaster hit on the rather happy device of giving him permission to wander off into the library during the classes. Alan looked at and later read books and picked up a good deal of haphazard information. This treatment led to the teacher developing a rather special relation with Alan, which made it difficult for the other masters. Alan took it as his right to behave with all the others as he behaved with his own class teacher, and thus he came to hold a unique position in the school, enhanced by the fact that he was regularly absent three times a week when he came for analytic treatment.

When the analysis ended the situation was better, in that Alan was more friendly towards other children and even collected a number of them round him, showing promise of becoming a leader; but he did not participate well in class work, and his educational attainment was patchy and mostly well below the average. How was this symptom to be managed?

When the hoped-for result from treatment with me had not materialized, the headmaster's tolerance became strained. Alan's presence in the school was an increasing source of anxiety and he could scarcely restrain his wish to expel the boy. Both Alan's parents fought for Alan to remain and his father produced penetrating arguments in his defence: he used my conclusion as to Alan's normality and pointed out the differences between Alan's behaviour at home and at school but, even with my support, he could not succeed. Because the headmaster could not believe Alan would respond to ordinary discipline, he wanted him moved to a school for maladjusted children. As Alan's parents' efforts were in serious danger of failing, I decided on active intervention.

Alan had by then become something of a *cause célèbre*, as will be apparent from the numerous people who were involved: Alan himself and his parents, his class teacher, his headmaster and the clinic staff, including myself. I invited all the contending parties to the clinic.

The conference centred on the headmaster's anxiety, which was sufficiently modified for him not to expel Alan from his school immediately. It was the group as a whole that achieved this result; my part was to draw out the various ideas that were being expressed, without giving much expression to my own views. When, for instance, Alan's supposed inaccessibility to discipline was made much of, doubts could be sown in the headmaster's mind by asking Alan's father to say what he had found, and then starting a discussion about the very different accounts. Other sources of anxiety centred on Alan's supposed 'intellectual subnormality' and on those aspects of Alan's achievements that showed promise. After some discussion, special tuition in a small group was suggested, and this seemed acceptable to all the group members; so the conference ended.

When Alan attended the small class, the teacher there soon began to find him brilliant and he began to learn rapidly. But still the headmaster continued to emphasize Alan's abnormal behaviour and to think of him as a blemish on his school.

Then a further crisis arose because his class teacher could not go on giving him special care: he was leaving the school, and Alan would therefore have to go to classes where he would meet other less skilled and tolerant teachers. This situation led to a second conference, and during it the headmaster's argument changed—he feared that with the less sensitive methods used by his class teachers Alan might be damaged beyond repair. Also, the headmaster did not believe the reports of Alan's intelligence and thought it out of the question for him to pass the eleven-plus (qualifying) examination and go to a grammar school, as the teacher giving him special tuition claimed was possible. The headmaster wanted further treatment at the clinic, suggesting that Alan would be made by me into a credit to his school. This I firmly resisted, for I believed it to be a danger signal; too often the attempt to shift responsibility onto somebody else leads to a child being kept at school only subject to his improving. As a consequence, teachers cease to exert themselves, and the next step is to say the child is not better, the treatment is not working and he is expelled. I suspected that the headmaster's request concealed this threat, so I asserted that Alan was able to adapt and held to this position so as to push the responsibility for failure back onto the teachers.

My idea was as follows: the balance between good and bad objects within Alan was decisively in favour of the good ones— this was maintained under the severe stress of ending his therapy and had gone over into his home; therefore there was a good prospect for a favourable change at school. Wherein lay the difficulty? On the one hand, there was a long history of special treatment, which Alan was not likely to relinquish easily. He had collected a store of unusual knowledge; it fascinated his class teacher but kept him outside class activities, other than those in which he could become a leader. On the other hand, because the masters had come to think of him as a special case, they did not give Alan a chance to become 'normal'. There was one step I had not so far taken. I did not believe that the earlier intelligence quotients were a correct estimate of Alan's present ability so I suggested that this was the time to re-test him. The headmaster capitulated and agreed to let Alan stay in his school so long as the test turned out as hoped for and so long as I would be prepared to treat him further if necessary. I readily agreed, but intended to resist it as long as possible. I was rather sure that it would not be necessary. The result of the test was an I.Q. of 120 with a scatter and some correct answers at superior adult level.

It was less easy to persuade the special teacher to relinquish the fascination that Alan had for her, but at length she did so, and later Alan was admitted to a grammar school, where he maintained himself successfully, and subsequently went to a University, studying mathematics and statistics at post-graduate level.

History

The following history was constructed from four sources: (a) the history collected at the first hospital, which Alan attended for about two years (it will be referred to as Hospital X); (b) some data provided in regular interviews with his mother during his analytic therapy, and (c) additional information provided at occasional interviews with father.

There resulted a number of different accounts, which often depended on how Alan's mother was feeling. I spent time evaluating them in relation to (d) information obtained from Alan's behaviour during his treatment.

FIRST FIVE MONTHS

Alan was a wanted baby and during pregnancy mother was healthy; the labour was short—five-and-a-half hours—and he weighed six pounds and six ounces. He was said to be a good, contented, happy baby, but 'not the cuddly type'. By this mother probably meant that breast-feeding for eight months went forward well and he took solids with pleasure, and became a big eater. There were no serious conflicts or sleep disturbances at the start, but he was not a passive good baby. His mother commented that besides the active feeding-pattern he did not cry much—a statement probably made in comparison with his later behaviour.

Alan was born with *talipes equinus*, and it may be significant that mother never made any comment on how she felt when she discovered the congenital defect; it usually comes as a shock.

FIVE TO FIFTEEN MONTHS

Treatment to correct the deformity of Alan's feet began round about three months when mother started taking him to hospital for massage. By five months she herself had taken over the treatment, which she had by then learnt how to administer: it included applying to his legs and feet Dennis Brown splints at night. These were said to become a centre of conflict with Alan, who would wake up 'screaming the place down', so that the splints 'had to be removed'. Father, who did not massage the feet or apply the splints, being more soft-hearted than mother, removed them more often than she did. Mother remarked once: 'When I put them on he took them off'—because, as he once said, 'I would rather have a child with a physical defect than with a mental disease'; and so 'as a tiny child Alan would always call for or turn to his father'.

As time went on, Alan became affectionate with him and loved being 'sung to and nursed by him'; details of when this developed were never given. It is difficult to evaluate this report because mother's guilt overlaid what she said, but it seems certain that there were ongoing conflicts in which Alan would scream, hit out, throw objects at mother and pull her hair. It is, I think, well to underline here that during at least three months (between five and eight months in terms of his age), when Alan's aggressive relation to his mother was developing, there was concurrently a good continuing relation over feeding. The two patterns persisted, though they were modified, as will be seen.

My quandary is this: from the way mother talked, there could be no doubt that she suffered; it is less certain that Alan did so. If his behaviour with me can be taken as referring to this period, pain would have been converted into aggression so quickly that suffering would not take place.

Distress over treatment of the talipes continued until Alan

was seventeen months old, when it was abandoned as a regular feature of his life. After a break, there followed intermittent attempts to apply the splints till the age of two and a half; from then on they were not used at all till he was three and a half. By then the right foot was normal and the left foot improving. By the time he started analytic therapy both feet were in effect normal.

It is rather tempting, when reviewing the management of the talipes, to think of the situation as sufficiently traumatic to be the main cause of his condition. This would be to agree with Alan's mother, who reproached herself for her bad and over-rigid management or failure to understand the 'psychological effects' of what she had done. No doubt the treatment must have caused discomfort and perhaps some physical pain as well, but not all babies who are treated thus become as aggressive as Alan. Aspects of the parents' style of upbringing may have been relevant here: mother was not a woman who showed her feelings easily in the interviews but made good contact in emotionally neutral or positive areas and was on the whole a warm thoughtful person. Both parents were given to losing their tempers and smacking the children, though they both hastened to add that they 'did not believe in it'! There was also an indicative observation made when Alan was at Hospital X: at the end of an interview, a note states, 'on the way out, when putting on Alan's coat, mother got hold of his arm, fairly shoving it into his sleeve, saying the while "Now say good morning to Miss 'C' ", which he did and then ran away.' This kind of rough behaviour over the splint was likely to have taken place at times when she was pre-occupied or exasperated, but I don't believe it would have been a regular feature of her behaviour. More significant was that mother's firmness was not supported by father and this would have given Alan a loophole to get rid of her. In this way, being an active baby anyway, he might have learned that aggressive screaming paid off. This hypothesis would explain the later use of aggression without restraint; a great deal of it could then be understood as getting rid of and triumphing over bad objects.

In other respects his mother thought of Alan's development as satisfactory, though his talking was rather late (it began at about two years and did not progress well). She once said that he had clean nappies before reaching his first birthday.

In view of the importance given in Alan's play to urine and faeces, in which anal sadism and passivity were very marked, it must be questioned whether clean nappies so early as one year was correct.

Mother's statements were indeed ambiguous; the early date was not stable and would shift to as late as fifteen months (she remembered that he controlled his bladder two months after walking at thirteen months). In addition, Alan suffered from attacks of diarrhoea that began between six and seven months and continued till $2\frac{1}{2}$ years (the date at which splints were discontinued), by which time he had become faecally incontinent again; it seems very unlikely that an infant with diarrhoea would always control his faeces. So how are we to understand this? Are we to rely on mother's distinction between incontinence and diarrhoea or not?

FIFTEEN TO EIGHTEEN MONTHS

Alan's parents thought it would be a good thing for them to have another baby: 'It might make things better'. Perhaps they thought Alan needed children of his own age, for they started him at nursery school rather early; the exact date is not known. Mother soon became pregnant and John was born when Alan was fifteen months old. Contrary to their hopes he 'took John's birth very badly', a statement that will be questioned. Most of the evidence for it was derived from some considerable time after the birth: indeed, not till he was three years old (cf. infra). Mother, however, made persistent efforts to put the change in Alan down to jealousy, though her conclusion often seemed strained and even theoretical; indeed it seemed too simple an explanation altogether, so we may consider what happened in detail.

Soon after the birth, the baby John started to vomit his food: it was found that he suffered from pyloric stenosis and two months after the birth mother and the baby went together to hospital. Alan was left with his father, who looked after him in the morning, before he went to work, and in the evening when he returned home; during the day Alan went to a nursery school. Father was very sure that his son suffered very much: he was no longer violent and aggressive but suffered 'internally'. This is my inference, but I do not see how father could have coped otherwise. Probably at the end of this period, so father told me, Alan became ill with influenza, though mother reported that it was conjunctivitis with recurrent colds. When mother returned she noticed a considerable change in her relation to Alan: she could not get in touch with him; as an instance of this she recorded that, whereas before, though he did not like cuddling, he would sit on her knee, now he would jump off whenever she put him there. This kind of inaccessibility continued, even though the aggressiveness returned.

Taking this period as a whole, Alan showed clear evidence of retreat and the most likely cause was a depression.

TWO YEARS

When he was two years old, Alan was taken, on and off, to a play group. At this time he also started an obsession about things being broken; there will be more about obsessions when considering the report of behaviour at Hospital X.

THREE YEARS

In the second half of his fourth year there seem to have been changes focusing on Christmas, when his grandparents were in the house; but it was also the time when the splints were started again (three and a half years). Once mother remarked that Alan did not show signs of jealousy till that Christmas; then he was three years eight months old. In this period she grouped a number of symptoms, which were related in her mind if not in reality: first there was Alan's refusal to eat because of visitors. Next, John (then aged 2 years 5 months) was not allowed to play with Alan's toys. Alan would refuse to include John in his prayers and once asserted: 'I'm John'; and if his splints were put on he would say: 'Put them on John'. A further feature of this period was a patch of dirty pants and renewed screaming. It was then that he stopped eating meat (especially liver).

Understanding all this as jealousy, mother once summed up by saying that Alan had not shown it at all when John was a baby but she was sure it was there, all bottled up. When saying this, she added that she had taken such a long time to recognize that it was jealousy; indeed it seems to have derived from a suggestion made during interviews at Hospital X.

Observations at Hospital X (between 3 years 10 months and 6 years 2 months).

When Alan was three years and ten months old, his parents were sufficiently concerned to seek specialist help at the hospital where he had been born. Alan was by then going to a play-centre and there had been complaints that he did not seem interested in the other children but threw things at them and sometimes hurt them. Mother said: 'He has always been a thrower and has broken many windows. He pulls hair and has violent outbursts of temper, which are quite sad to see because he seems overcome by them.' Another concern of hers was that he dwelt on 'macabre things', a remark that she did not develop further.

It may have been noticed that so far very little that was positive emerged from mother's account of her son. She sometimes, however, implied good potential when she said he could talk 'if he wanted to'. In one positive statement, she did say he was very good with his hands, especially at taking things to pieces. At that time, she also reported that he loved engines, and father often took him to St. Pancras Station to look at them. He also had a passion for water-pipes and always pointed them out to mother. These observations were in contrast to her more general view that he did not seem interested in anybody or anything. There were various indications that his lack of positive attachment to her had made her resentful and jealous of his relation to his father; or it may have been for this reason that she had difficulty in assembling good characteristics. In the context of these observations, she also remarked how he was fond of men and very attached to his father.

In the first interview at Hospital X, mother referred to Alan's 'masturbation', which she subsequently described: 'He jumps up and down on the bed, his face becomes flushed and he gets much enjoyment therefrom.'

It also appeared that he then had periods of not eating; this was mentioned once again in relation to visitors or being away from home, but there was also a note to say that after attending play-therapy for a short time mother commented that he was eating a lot better—so difficulties with food may have been more general. It is conceivable that this was due to disturbance of his routine, for later he developed a ritual round food times. There seem to have been other obsessional characteristics, for

247

at this time he was said to get into terrible states if he was not allowed to do things in his own particular way.

In the second series of intelligence tests he showed a pre-occupation with numbers and an apparently compulsive tendency to give the wrong answers, which he then denied repeating the process as though it were a ritual. Also at 4 years 9 months, mother reported rituals over dressing, e.g. if mother put his socks on before his pants he was very upset.

Speech

In view of his tendency (very marked in the first psychiatric interview at Hospital X) to repeat questions and answers three or more times, interpreted as magic thinking, the state of his verbal knowledge and capacity to communicate were gone into He did not talk much but could talk in sentences; mother thought he could talk but would not. He muttered and whispered to himself and may have been developing a private language. He never used the first person and would repeat phrases and questions. In spite of these defects, speech was apparently adequate during the play-therapy for there were no comments on it.

There were interesting indications at this time that he was thinking about his feet; he would often point to his foot and say 'broken' and became interested in the picture of a pixie's foot that we turned up, remarking that this was broken. This led to mother recognizing that he thought about his feet and this may have been related to her earlier remarks about 'psy-chology'.

Jealousy of John was also referred to at Hospital X. The evidence given was once again not very strong, though mother seemed quite sure that there was jealousy. At 4 years 9 months, mother reported that Alan would suddenly hurl himself on John; there were also some rather strained efforts to interpret bits of symbolic behaviour in terms of jealousy.

Destructiveness (4 years 3 months)

On one occasion he very quickly cut up mother's tartan slacks and after this mother said she felt Alan's destructiveness was 'morbid' and 'sadistic': he seemed to enjoy destruction for its own sake. That Alan was enjoying being destructive was confirmed in his play sessions at Hospital X: he enjoyed trying to pull off the head and arms and legs of a doll and he commented with pleasure on a doll without a head and without a toe. He tried to break a toy motor-car by hitting the bumper and the idea of eating a girl doll was felt as pleasurable; 'She's nice to eat', he said. All this was recorded in a single note when Alan was 4 years 10 months. On this and on other occasions there was thumb-sucking, pleasure in making messes, much interest in water-taps and plug-holes and provocative throwing of water on the floor. The play-therapist thought that much of this play (e.g. *throwing* water on the floor or wiping dirty hands on her skirt to make her angry) was provocative and that he was not always just destructive, especially as he made efforts at reparation: given a doll with detachable head, arms and legs, he pulled them off and then spent some time rearticulating them.

In the report there are accounts of Alan's violent behaviour in public—in a bus, for instance, when there was not a place for him to sit beside his mother. At four years and eleven months, she reported, he had fears at night and difficulties in going to sleep; she then found that it helped if she got into bed with him until he went to sleep. He would also wake up at night and come into his parents' bed; and he would dream of an aeroplane or that bears got into his room.

Birth of Third Baby, Christopher

While Alan was having treatment at Hospital X, his parents were wanting to have a third baby but were deterred by anxiety lest Alan reacted as violently to the birth of the third child as he did to the second, even though what happened after the birth was not made clear; another contributing factor may have been that there had been a miscarriage. However, Alan's parents eventually went ahead with it. There is no mention in my notes about how this was taken, except that shortly after Christopher was born Alan used to talk to himself in bed, saying how he hated the baby.

About five months later, Alan made a rag doll—a boy called Grete—and everything that mother did for the baby Alan insisted on doing for Grete. This was a mixed identification with mother, who treated the baby well, and his father, who had also done this for Alan. Thus he found a way of being good to Christopher; he seems often to have achieved it. Mother thought that Grete might be Alan and tried to make approaches, thinking he was wanting affection but met with no response; she 'could not get near him at all'. This is the only mention of anything like a transitional object.

Then again one day Alan—during my treatment—was being very slow at getting into bed and mother shouted at him. He hit the baby, making her even more furious; she told Alan to put on his pyjamas and then she would come to him. When she went into the bedroom she found the baby in bed and Alan had his arms round him, cuddling him; he said: 'I only hit him because you were angry with me'. On another occasion, John interfered with the baby and mother told him to stop; Alan kicked John in the face, mother pulled him away so he threw a slipper at his brother.

In the end, mother seems to have come to the conclusion that Alan was mothering Christopher, for there was a comment: 'Alan has stopped arguing with the baby and is quite motherly with him again'.

Summary and Interpretation

It seems quite clear that in the first five months Alan and his mother formed a good basis for further development to proceed. I assume that this persisted so that a good mother was known to exist.

At five months, treatment of Alan's talipes began. His screaming could be thought of as the healthy response of an aggressive baby and it is also possible that in the first place the screaming was not due to the splints.

We know that by five months the infant has established object-relations based on omnipotence, that his objects are predominantly self-objects in the sense that there is a fusion between external objects and self-representations. This means there are 'fantastic images', i.e., that he is liable to react with terror to the generation of images or events that may seem insignificant to somebody else.

The period at which splints were applied may have been unfortunate, for Mahler conceives that the height of symbiosis is reached between the fourth and fifth month and it is at about this time that Klein held that there were signs of pining, i.e., the onset of the depressive position. Thus the splints may have been applied at a period of crisis in Alan's maturation and it could have been that anxieties were focused on the splints by Alan's parents. Each of them had a style of living that included aggression, and it was basically of the safe kind, and this would be one reason why Alan's aggression was not driven back on him; but it is probable that, if mother had become angry, the baby would have been frightened; in addition she had compulsive trends that may have made her inflexible and rough.

However she behaved, and even if his waking at night and screaming was not due to discomfort caused by the splints, we may safely assume that here is the root of Alan's fantasy of a good breast-mother and a bad witch-mother. It would, however, have been basically part of healthy development, had not father stepped in and undermined mother's efforts at treatment; thus he may have reinforced and confused the situation: who is the good mother? Here would be the basis for the later reversed oedipal pattern.

Alan's father was so much Alan's ally that he only had to scream loudly enough for him to arrive and give comfort and for the splints to be removed. Since the pattern of aggressive discharge continued for years, it seems that this was the root of the discovery that violence paid off (reinforcement of manic defences). Thus, one pattern of Alan's life was formed in which a basically persecutory situation was converted into triumph over the bad mother, which his real mother could become should the real father contain all the good-mother attributes. Diarrhoea started at 6-7 months, soon after the splints were applied. It may have been a technique. Alan's body was used to eject his rage, which was already characterized by its respiratory 'incontinence' (screaming) and hitting out. To assume this is not to deny its additional association with teething.

We can now approach the birth of John and the absence of his mother when she went into hospital with the baby; this was followed by Alan becoming inaccessible to his mother. My inference is that Alan became depressed and had not recovered from it by the time he came for analytic therapy—I suppose that he has never done so completely.

Neither of his parents recognized the change as such but father was deeply moved by it and mother put it down to jealousy of the baby. But was it? Or was the mother's reconstruction a displacement of her own jealousy? In the first place, the advent of the baby coincided with a temporary end to his treatment, which mother could not apply and father would not —he preferred 'a child with a physical defect rather than a mental illness'; so this could be thought of as a triumph for Alan. Bearing in mind the nature of omnipotence, however, the triumph of his aggression would mean the death of his bad witch-mother and, because of his regression, of the good one too. How, then can it be understood that the birth of John made no impact? The answer comes from further reflection on omnipotence. It is not a stage in which such a sophisticated experience as jealousy can be felt. Mother's idea that he felt it inside him presupposes that Alan had an inside where it could be lodged. From what is known of Alan this was not so. So we need to look for alternative explanations. In omnipotence an event can easily be treated as non-existent by negative hallucination, in which case the painful situation is done away with: this is very much in line with how Alan treated painful situations. It involves, however, an increase in destructive affects directed towards his mother. As there was already a predisposition to treat his mother as bad, through transfer of her good attributes to the father, a situation fraught with danger arose and, when mother disappeared, the feeling that she was dead could come over him with total violence.

But why was it that he could not manage this as a triumph over the bad mother? There were two factors here: first, his father left him for much of the day and he had to cope with the nursery school, so he could not really use him as a good mother; next, in his development he had experienced his own mother as a good one. He could not transfer the good mother to the father because he went away too much and left him with strangers. Therefore, by regression, the absent good mother had gone (was dead). He might have pined, but he did not; he could not and so depression replaced pining, sadness and grief, which were not known to him.

Then there is the fact that all the evidence for Alan's being jealous derives from late in his third year. It seems that Alan was hitting John, hiding his toys, throwing objects about, breaking windows and other things for a long time before this, but there are only phrases like 'he has always been a thrower' to support such an idea of an earlier origin for jealousy. Could it have been that the link with his earlier aggressive and relatively more healthy period was re-established soon after the splint was re-applied regularly at $3\frac{1}{2}$ years of age? There was also a bout of diarrhoea, which would support the notion. We are on uncertain ground; there seems, however, no doubt that a change of some sort took place and that it was rather to do with Alan himself than with any environmental influence. At first sight it might be blamed on 'stranger anxiety' and I would not exclude this, especially as he was sent to strangers when mother went into hospital.

Another suggestive event was this: it will be remembered that a considerable change took place at home in the relation between Alan and his parents soon after treatment began. Whereas before the oedipal situation had been reversed, it soon became altered. Alan hated his father and loved his mother.

Could it not have been that the taking up of Alan's *pre*-oedipal conflicts in the transference released libido and aggression for a development that had begun and could now proceed? If this were so, then the disturbance at 3 years 6 months was due to the maturation of oedipal patterns, which Alan could not cope with because of the genital excitement this brought to the fore and complex emotional demands that were laid on his ego.

Obsessional Characteristics

There remains the manifestation of obsessional characteristics: rituals over dressing, over food, signs of obsessions over numbers; and, it will be remembered, the structuring in a ritualistic manner of his interviews with me described in Part Three. Thus it would seem that he tried to use obsessional defences but later discarded them.

APPENDIX

INTELLIGENCE TESTS ON ALAN

Test 1. Date: 19.6.56

Date of birth   24.4.52
Test used   Merrill-Palmer scale
General results   C.A. = 50 months (4 years, 2 months)
       M.A. = 36 months (3 years)
       Percentile rank = between 5-19 (inferior)
       Sigma value = —.2.0

BEHAVIOUR: Alan was slightly hesitant to come with me. He refused to look at me or to leave his chair but, with a slight persuasion, he agreed with his mother to come and see the pictures with me in another room.

In the testing room he showed no anxiety. He was compliant and settled down in his chair rather submissively. He was co-operative but did not apply himself well to the tasks. He lacked persistence and tended to look away, while sucking his first two fingers vigorously. At those moments he looked very babyish and tended to close his eyes also.

He always started with his left hand but used both in between the tasks.

He was rather passive and made no attempt to leave his chair even when we had finished.

RESULTS: The scale suggests that Alan is below average in intelligence, but he did not seem to be using his potentiality to the full and showed inconsistent performance. His motor control was not very good. Although his perception for figure and ground was accurate, he made little attempt to fit the pieces in their spaces properly and completed the task only with constant encouragement. He could not button, or move his thumb while closing his fist.

His speech is not very clear but he was able to answer questions and repeat groups of words.

SUMMARY: Alan seems to be a boy of below average intelligence. His general behaviour was rather babyish and he showed motor immaturity but there were indications, however, that he was not using his potentiality to the full and must be tested again after some time.

Test 2. Date: 11.4.58

BEHAVIOUR: Alan looks like a six-year-old; in behaviour he was less immature than when last tested. The finger-sucking and dreamy, withdrawn expression were not in evidence today.

Some of his reactions seemed to be very defensive, scribbling over work he had done, writing numbers instead of drawing what he was asked to draw, etc. There was an air of provocation about him when doing these things, but he seemed to me a very disturbed child and not so much one who was testing out an adult.

TEST FINDING: REVISED STANFORD-BINET, FORM L.

C.A. = 5 years 11 months;
M.A. = 5 years 2 months;
I.Q. = 87

Note: This contains a high rote memory success, without which the I.Q. would be 82, i.e., very little change from last time.

A boy of inferior intelligence. He does better in verbal, memory and number items. His attention to pictorial and perceptual material is fitful, his response impulsive. He seems to have the goodwill to try whatever he is asked but withdraws his effort in a most unpredictable way.

There is an element of stereotypy in his response and some perseveration.

General Comment

Alan seems to have a drive to achievement and an awareness of his inadequacies that, combined, are very burdensome. He is preoccupied with numbers and writes them out rapidly as if in a frenzy. He wrote out spontaneously various number-combinations, e.g. $2 + 1 =$, traced over the figures again and again, repeated the problem several times before adding an answer and sometimes seemed to give compulsively a wrong answer, which he then denied, repeating the process as though it were a ritual. Evidently he is encouraged in these activities and perhaps even pressed.

School must find him a problem in behaviour and difficult to understand.

AGE: Ten years, five months.   Dates: 9.10.61 and 16.10.62.
TESTS: 1. Revised Stanford-Binet, Form L.
            Mental age 12 years 6 months at least
            I.Q. 120
         2. Schonell's Mechanical Arithmetic
            Arithmetic age 12 years 9 months
         3. Schonell's Reading Vocabulary
            Reading age 12 years 1 month
         4. Schonell's Silent Reading B.
            Reading age 13 years

Comments:

Alan is in fact a child of above average intelligence. His I.Q. may well be an under-estimate since he was so anxious to do well that his concentration on what he was doing was sometimes impaired by his anxiety about the next, or the previous, problem.

On educational tests his reading and arithmetic ages are at least two years in advance of his chronological age. He writes quite swiftly and fairly legibly, but his writing is clumsy with very heavy pressures and resembles that of a child of under ten. He seemed to enjoy putting things in writing, however, and spontaneously sat down at the end of the test and wrote out a story about a ghost, making it up as he went along.

Analysis of his successes and failures on the Binet suggest that he is a child of verbal rather than non-verbal, or performance, ability. He failed two performance tests (memory for design and paper-cutting) at the nine-year level, but passed reasoning tests at the Average Adult and Superior Adult level.

He was fidgety and talked a great deal (relevantly) during the Intelligence test, but he settled down quite well to Reading and Arithmetic tests, which he worked by himself. His speech is a little indistinct—for example, he mixes up some consonants, saying *l* for *r*, etc., and talks fast and abruptly. He also has a tic, in which he draws up his upper lip every few seconds.

He made good contact with me and, although clearly anxious about his performance and wanting to be assured that he had done well, he appeared to enjoy coping with intellectual problems.

Alan is a child who is certainly capable of working at a grammar school standard, but he needs a good deal of individual attention if he is to produce anything like his best work, and he should be taught in as small a group as possible.

JAMES

Introduction

I have selected James for study because he was an autistic child whose prognosis was unfavourable. Speech was virtually absent at the age of eight when I started to see him. His autism 'appeared' in the course of an otherwise even development, though it must have been there before it was discovered. He was an easy baby and his mother did not observe anything to cause anxiety until he failed to talk.

I wanted to test my ideas about autism, which I thought might be a disorder of integration and might represent the persistence of the primary self that had prevented the infant relating to his mother at the start. That there were no bouts of screaming, crying or other signs of distress during the breast-feeding period suggested that the integration was unusually complete and that the baby did not feel the effect of inevitable frustrations, nor did he give evidence of passing through the crisis periods in early development. I wanted, when I treated him, to create conditions under which the primary integrate could be reached, and to provide opportunities for James to take the initiative in coming into relation with me, rather than my making a relation with him. I did not know how to create these conditions and as I went along with him I adopted other ideas about how to treat an autistic child, because I wanted to see if I could 'help' him without violating my basic premise. I shall record the methods I adopted, as I describe the various changes and developments that took place. Throughout, I was concerned to put to the test my original idea, which made me consistently relate to what seemed to come from him and to stop any activity on my part that caused distress or puzzlement in him.

In the case-description I have given details of his behaviour and changes in it. This has made a comparatively short account of a relation that lasted for seven years. The brevity of it is due to months of repetitive activity, which did not change in any essential respect. During these fallow periods I asked myself over and over again whether there was any sense in continuing to see him; but then some change would take place that gave a ray of hope and it was supported by both James and his parents, who were keen to go on and attended with great regularity, though I had consistently refused to hold out hopes of benefit.

In looking over my notes some years after I had stopped seeing James, I was surprised by the developments that had taken place. His case had, by the end, induced a depressive countertransference that interfered with an assessment of what had been achieved. I must have known about this somewhere, but it took me a long time before I could see it at all clearly.

History

James's birth was said to be normal and he was breast-fed for nine months, during which time his mother could remember nothing unusual. He was at first neither lazy nor aggressive, he sucked vigorously without ever biting the breast, in fact everything went smoothly; the account was, however, slightly modified by one remark: his mother fed him regularly on a four-hourly routine that she adapted to 'crises', so presumably there were difficulties. As an example, she said that when James woke up at night on four occasions she fed him then, but this hardly seemed to warrant her use of such a dramatic word.

Weaning was attempted at about six months, when James's mother tried to see whether he would take one or two solid foods, using a spoon; he rejected the food and she did not press him to eat. When he was about eight months old she gave him Farex, again using a spoon. Finding that he liked this and enjoyed his feed she continued with it and gradually transferred him to other solids without difficulty. He quickly came to use the spoon himself.

The feeding history was gone into with care, twice; each time the account was essentially the same. It is in marked contrast to the account given by others, that autistic children suffer from feeding difficulties, sometimes severe, with ritualistic testing of food by the child as if it were dangerous.

The only symptoms belonging to this period were felt by the mother in herself. She had been married for ten years when James was born; she wanted him, though her husband was not so keen. He was a regular officer in the Royal Air Force and had been shot down twice over Germany during World War II, but got back to England with the help of the Resistance movement. He was finally killed, and his wife was informed of his death, five days before James's birth. She was 'upset and nervous' during the breast-feeding; even this admission was uncharacteristic of a woman who hid or repressed her feelings and emotions: she never once mentioned being sad or depressed by her husband's death. As I shall detail later, she showed evidence of an obsessional character-structure, and it is quite possible that she did not, indeed could not, mourn her husband's death, but only felt compelled to ward off a depression at the time. If this conclusion is correct, then her depression would have been a decisive factor in her relation to her baby. In other words, there is support here for the idea that the origin of autism derives from premature induction of the depression in the baby.

James's teething was late, beginning at about fifteen months, and it presented no problems; the process might not have caused any feelings inside the child's mouth at all.

The first symptom that caused any concern was backwardness. James did not walk until he was two or more and he never wanted to crawl. His mother offered a reason for the late walking: she said that her son would do a thing when he was ready for it and would not do anything until he could do it well—this applied to his walking, which he learnt rapidly once he made the effort to do so.

Training in sphincter control was not attempted until James walked, and was established as follows. When mother's second husband (whom she married a year after James's birth) was away from home in the summer she let James wander about with scarcely any clothes on; she kept her eye on him and led him to the pot whenever he seemed to want to urinate or defaecate. He was clean in ten days. In this connection, mother remarked that he had been smacked on two occasions so that he must have done something 'naughty', but what this was she did not tell.

Talking has never developed, though it began; his first words were 'wee wee' and 'lav' and he seems to mouth words and even sentences now (i.e. at eight years old), but no sounds come out of his mouth at these times. Because of the delay in his speech he was taken to a neurologist who referred him for speech training, and this was continued after I saw him. It led to no improvement in speech, though at first his mother felt it was helpful: she reported that the therapist sat James on her knee and cuddled him for some of the time.

James had only one illness—measles, when he was three years old. He was nursed at home and there were no complications.

By eight years of age his play was restricted to mechanical exercises; he liked toys that take to pieces and can be put together again. For a short period there had been a brief spell of aggressive play: he broke up his toys but his mother told him it was 'naughty'; this was sufficient to control him and the behaviour stopped.

He did not play with other children but liked to watch them, especially if they were playing with his toys. As an only child, he had therefore been in the company of his parents for most of the time.

The overall picture given by this history is of an unassertive child, who seems to have conformed all along to a passive behaviour pattern. Apart from the negative symptom of retarded development, the mother reported nothing else at the outset.

Soon after treatment began, another facet of his home life was added: before treatment began he had been restless and mother had been forced to say 'don't' to him 'all the time'. This negative picture was incomplete: there were positive features in his relation to his mother—for instance, he helped her in various ways in the house, particularly in washing-up.

1. Parents' Personalities

Mother was an extremely capable, controlling woman who could be direct, determined and forceful. This showed in her efforts to get James to a school, her primary aim when she first brought him to the clinic. It also appeared when she dealt with the educational authorities, who enquired about James's absence from school. Then she became very outspoken and vigorous in her denunciation of them; she could be equally determined in her handling of her son and her husband.

A very marked feature of her relations with the clinic was her persistence in bringing James. She controlled his coming and going like a machine; they were never late and, though I asked her not to influence James's behaviour in the clinic, she could not bring herself to stop. It would be wrong to say she lacked affect, but if possible she always converted it into action; this gave the impression that she could tolerate neither tender nor loving feeling nor fantasy. Indeed, during almost the whole period covered by her interviews with the psychiatric social worker, she never said anything personal or intimate, though it sometimes looked as if she was near crying. For quite a long time she developed one persistent idea: that we were wanting her to let James destroy her home, knowing how important it was to her. This presumably was what she felt would happen if she relaxed control of James and perhaps of herself also.

The point I am driving at is this: given a compliant depressive trend in James, he could have been exploited by his mother to produce a picture not unlike that given by her. She often talked about her child as if he were an animal and she gave the impression of training him with the sort of firmness which is useful in animal training.

But she was capable of and made very great sacrifices. Bringing her son to the clinic was one, and there were others, but I may perhaps best illustrate what I mean by describing a single event. There had been difficulties with her second husband, whose irascible nature was getting the better of him, and James was acting in such a way as to bring it out. Matters reached a climax and mother said she would sell up the house, and she and James would go off together without her husband if he did not control his temper. This incident had complex implications, but whatever the relation between her and her husband, which was never gone into in any detail, they formed a very effective combination in numerous respects.

James's stepfather was accepted by James as his father. Apart from his tempers, he was a retiring man and was said by his wife to be nervy; but he was the more emotional of the two and could express affection and anger, particularly the latter.

James would, according to his mother when she first came to the clinic, drive his stepfather into a frenzy, which made the child panic-stricken; she would always protect her son from it—the incident over the house illustrates how.

One feature that remained constant throughout the time that James came to the clinic was the remarkable affective un-communicativeness of both parents, which gave the impression that they were basically isolated, though in an adapted obsessional manner. I was drawn to take particular notice of their behaviour and I will record one piece of it as worthy of being detailed because it suggests the significance of James's interest in clocks, very marked at the time. The behaviour was much the same for each parent, but I could observe it best with the stepfather because he regularly parked his car on the opposite side of the road from the clinic, where I could see him.

During James's interview he would sit in the car reading a book, then just when the interview was ending he would look at his watch, shut his book, get out of his car, walk across the road and meet James as he came out of the clinic. With very few exceptions, their arrival at the clinic entrance synchronized. It was as if this bit of behaviour, and perhaps much more, had been controlled by an internal clock and they were the instruments of it. This behaviour probably stemmed from James's mother, who also behaved like this when not coming to see the psychiatric social worker. At first father simply sat in his car and James ran across the road, but this stopped suddenly when mother discovered what was happening.

2. A Description of James before Treatment

So as to give a suggestion of how James appeared before treatment began, I cannot do better than extract the excellent description given by the psychologist during her interview with James. When he was 5 years and 3 months old he was seen in the presence of students. She says: 'James came with me from the waiting-room without demur, and at his mother's suggestion I took him by the hand. His hand was cool, limp and entirely unresponsive. He was busy exploring his surroundings visually, turning his head about, looking at doors, windows, stairs, passages.

'In my room he settled in a chair for a few minutes, doing the three-figure-board, but after that failed to respond in any way to myself or to the students. I provided him with the toy material of the Revised Stanford-Binet Scale (cars, engines, cups, spoons, a fork, a chain, small girl doll, cats, a dog).

'He did not "play" with these, but he became entirely absorbed in arranging and re-arranging the cars, cups, spoons, and fork and chain into a neat, compact group, the cars lined up side by side, the two cups together. The toys seemed to have no meaning to him, except as objects to be arranged. The one exception was the doll; he tried to make it stand, looked at its feet, turned up its skirt to examine the body. One arm came off by accident. He pulled off the other arm and spent much time trying, neatly and deftly, to replace the arms.

'He made occasional inarticulate sounds and when a student rolled cars towards him on the floor, or hid small objects in the palm of his hand, James showed pleasure by smiling and chuckling. But his pleasure seemed to be in the moving object, or in the recovering of an object, and not in playing with the student. Throughout he disregarded the people in the room and occupied himself entirely with inanimate objects, which he handled gently and deftly.

'At first we considered the possibility of his being deaf, but he responded just as little to touch and gesture as to the spoken word'.

This description fits in very well with a diagnosis of autism: the child's interest in objects and lack of response to people, as if they did not exist except, so it seemed, as part of a mechanical world that could be manipulated. It was as if his affect was thin, superficial and gave no meaning to what was done. To put it differently, the activities gave the impression that there was no person acting. James soon showed this characteristic in his interviews with me: when he wanted me to do something with my hand, he would take hold of it and treat it as if it were a bit of machinery.

Another feature was his limp unresponsive hand, part of his passive compliance. It may have been that his rapid toilet training came about because he complied with his mother's intentions, rather than wanting to become clean and control his excreta in his own way.

Intermixed with this very compliant pattern of behaviour,

autistic children usually exhibit occasional violent outbursts. James had not shown them at home before coming to the clinic.

The contrast between the psychologist's report and his mother's is very striking. She gave very little picture of what her child was like, and even taking into account differences in descriptive skill, the mother's account is almost entirely lacking in empathy. Yet the style of her upbringing was clever, tolerant and resourceful.

The most striking feature in her story was an absence. Imagine a healthy pregnant mother whose husband's life was recurrently in danger; one day he did not return, he was missing, he returned after a month's anxiety. This happened more than once, but five days before the baby was born he was killed. All this was bad enough but a mother would surely have emotions about it and be able to express what she went through. James's mother could not do this: she seemed not to be the kind of person to express emotions or to work through them. She managed well and was the sort of person who evokes admiration, but the repressed depression underneath may have made empathy impossible. So it is possible to reconstruct an early development in which her baby would be made to fit into her competence, in which there is, however, no room for it to develop a self-representation, since his mother does not see him as a person; through her own affective depletion, she sees him like an animal, to be trained.

TREATMENT

The First Period

At first James was very abstracted; he did not seem to notice or hear anything. I talked to him about my being a bad person and told him I thought he felt there was good inside him. I drew pictures illustrating my idea; at first he took little notice, but gradually became less abstracted and paid attention to the dolls' house. He touched it repeatedly, looked into it, took the front off, arranged the furniture in order and put little figures sitting round a table. One person was put in a bed and some were arranged against the walls. The mother was always put downstairs. After this he put the front back and repeatedly looked inside, as if to see whether everything was all right. A prominent feature was his care in making sure that all the doors between rooms were shut.

When I talked about the insides of people, following up his taking the front of the dolls' house off, and about possible dangers there, he became aggressive and pulled objects, pictures and a fireplace off the walls; he was especially interested in the bed, which he took out and tried to break up. Before going away he put all the objects back, except one—the toy fireplace, which he threw into a box of bricks in the play-room. Three interviews later (three weeks, for I saw him once a week) he sought it out and put it back in the dolls' house. Once, after putting the front back, he placed a little woolly animal in the front door.

Other activities were his dancing approach to and tendency to look underneath objects, such as the furniture. He repeatedly took off the baby doll's clothes and inspected its buttocks; once he pulled off the detachable arm. He finished this activity by putting the doll in a perambulator, which he wheeled away into the corner. In these activities he would smile and look delighted; periodically he would suck his fingers and slobber with his mouth.

He became interested in taking toy cars to pieces, and several times he threw one up in the air and watched it fall and break. When this happened he tried to mend it and used my hand as an apparatus to help in typical autistic fashion. There seemed no distress over the breakage.

For a short time he introduced a barrier into his activities: he crowded my toys together behind a row of fences.

At first James treated me as though I were not there, but he seemed to respond to what I said; he avoided looking at me. During this period, I told him he felt I was dangerous and concurrently I tried various activities to see what he would do. I offered him a four-coloured pencil from my pocket—he put it down on the table; I could lightly pat the table to make a noise and he laughed. Once I turned on the water-tap in the sink. He seemed to take no notice but later on he went and looked at it. After that, if I came close to him, he would occasionally inspect and touch my face. When I developed a playful game of attacking him, he retaliated by pinching and squeezing my cheeks. As time went on, he approached me and even took the pencil I had offered him out of my pocket, encouraged me to draw and scribble and patted my face on the cheek, and became interested in a mole on my upper lip, which he seemed keen to remove in a mechanical fashion.

Improvement at Home

Before he started treatment he had been restless and difficult at home so that his mother was 'always having to say *no*'. He had, however, a number of occupations, like taking objects to pieces and putting them together; he used Triang toys, picture puzzles and picture books, and liked television. If taken to meet other children, or if they were invited to his home, he would watch them playing with apparent pleasure but never joined in.

About three months after treatment started, mother reported a number of improvements. She found him easier to manage. He was less restless and settled to sustained activities. He carried out her orders intelligently, ran his own bath and undressed himself; he laid the table for lunch correctly. He began to make more sounds like words: 'Nnn', for instance, like the beginning of 'No'; he could say 'Yes', and four months later he said: 'Mummy'. He imitated consonants 'm-m', 'b-b-b' and 'k-k-k' and added three words: 'tea', 'home', 'scissis'.

Occasionally he had become mischievous; for instance, he transplanted mother's plants and started doing things to annoy her, breaking out into laughter when she became angry. He started to develop his relations with others and he even went on his own to play with a neighbour's child of about three years. These and other changes encouraged James's mother and she did not send him to the Rudolf Steiner School, as she had intended, making a condition, however, that I would see him twice a week, which I did.

Hide-and-Seek Activities

This first phase lasted about one year, during which some progress had been made. Then, influenced by the idea that effort was needed to draw the autistic child out of his isolation, I dramatized his isolation by starting a game of hiding behind a screen, pretending I was frightened. At first he took no notice; next he came and pulled me out of my hiding place and later adopted my style of behaviour by hiding himself somewhere.

This developed into an elaborate hide-and-seek activity, which became difficult to manage.

At this time, the clinic had been housed in a flat on the first floor; there was another vacant one on the same floor. Downstairs was a psychiatric clinic for adult patients and on the floor above was another vacant flat. Thus there were a number of rooms into which James's activities could expand without there being a demonstrable reason why particular rooms should not be used. The clinic rooms, in which interviews were being conducted, were naturally taboo and so there were places, besides the adult clinic downstairs, to which he could not be allowed free access. This state of affairs became important when James started to escape from the play-room and run round the passage and other rooms in the clinic, one of which was regularly vacant; but he could enter the lavatory and the secretary's room because she was a tolerant, interested person.

At first I let him run about but then, to restrict his activities, I would introduce frustrations, stopping him going out of the room, for instance. This did not work very well because he would sometimes fight quite hard to push past me. I did not resist much, furthermore there were two exits to the play-room; if I did succeed in preventing him going out of either door he started throwing objects out of the window. When I tried to stop this, too, he could draw me away from the doors and slip out of the room, so throwing objects away became a thought-out trick. I therefore changed my behaviour and started going round the rooms with him. Again he would escape, hiding in a cupboard or locking himself in the lavatory for quite a long time. I dealt with this by finding him when he hid in a cupboard or waiting for him if he had gone into the lavatory, from which he would eventually emerge.

James liked being found and it became possible to develop a hide-and-seek activity in which one would hide and the other seek. Sometimes the game became quite hilarious, especially if I was 'hiding' and then appeared from an unexpected direction. I tried to restrict his activities to the first clinic floor and if he went down or upstairs I would bring him back by holding his hand, putting my arm round him or jumping him up the stairs with both my arms round him, or even carrying him on my shoulders, so that quite close physical contacts were established. But more important was the inevitable distinction made between places that were allowed, and those that were forbidden. This he clearly understood, and if he went into a forbidden place, like the stairs to the ground floor, and I did not fetch him back, he would make a noise by stamping until I did so; again, if he went into the room where his mother was being interviewed —at one time he did this regularly—and I did not remove him, he looked disappointed, sad and dejected.

It was most striking that much of this activity was like that of a normal child who might be mentally defective. He never, however, spoke a word, and there were definitely autistic features in that he would peer into dark places, which I called 'dark mummy' or would have periods of wandering round abstracted and 'lost'. Often when I frustrated him physically he would exhibit signs of passive compliance but this could be converted fairly easily into a tug-of-war game.

Without doubting the diagnosis of autism, therefore, the play might suggest additional mental retardation. Clinically there did not seem much other evidence to support the idea, and intelligence tests indicated the contrary, though it is of course difficult to get good evidence without co-operation. The first test, when James was seven, and before treatment had started, suggested that he was 'at least average non-verbal intelligence', but co-operation in the tests was minimal. A second test one year later, about seven months after treatment had begun, and in which co-operation was very much better, gave the astonishing I.Q. of 160 for Koh's blocks and 146 for the Alexander Passalong Test.

During this period James developed an activity that was to persist. He started chewing the thenar eminence of his right hand, and developed a callosity there that was still present when I stopped seeing him. Chewing activity was often related to external frustration and would sometimes start in periods of internal stress such as before initiating some activity to which he could not foresee my reaction, but there often seemed little reason for it. The chewing may have been related to interpreting his fear of my eating him up but there was no very clear connection. By contrast, when I held him he would from time to time get hold of bits of my skin and twist them fiercely; he did not persist and I did not have to stop him. Later on he developed these physical attacks to some extent.

It was in relation to my stopping his extra-clinic activities that he began to shut me out of the play-room, pushing me through the entrance and then shutting the door and resisting my coming in again.

After eighteen months' treatment, James reacted to my going away on holiday for three weeks. His mother reported deterioration in his behaviour. She was in tears, a quite astonishing state for her to reveal, because she felt that James had got out of control. She said he had not settled to any occupation, and she had felt compelled to go back to 'watching him all the time'. He wandered about the house banging doors and stamping, turning off gas-taps, tearing up magazines, scribbling on books, dropping pencils down the lavatory, and he started wandering off and she did not know where he might not go.

After I came back, James once more became amenable to her influence and, with support, she succeeded in managing one piece of behaviour skilfully. While I was away he had started to spread his food on the tablecloth, and to wipe his knife and fork on it. After talking this over with the social worker she tore up a sheet, let him eat in the kitchen and do as he liked; the behaviour gradually stopped.

When I saw James again he was unusually apprehensive about his mother. Before she went for her interview, and while she was sitting in the waiting-room, he left the treatment-room door open, crouched down on the floor, or looked out with a puzzled, worried look. As soon as he was sure his mother had departed for her interview or had left the clinic, he began his usual activities, at first restricting them to the clinic, though soon he began departing to other 'forbidden' places.

As the excursions did not seem productive, and as my presence was by now clearly important, I decided to stay in the room until James came back to 'find' me, which he began to do. He then developed rejecting activities. He would take objects out of my pockets and if I objected would struggle to get them, laughing and emitting high-pitched squeaks and gurgles; he started pushing me out of the door and shut it with a bang—the noise was important, for if I prevented it he would insist on its being made. Concurrently he developed his earlier activity of throwing objects out of the window in large numbers, and this seemed so important that I let him do it, collecting the toys afterwards. Eventually he focused on the baby doll and I tied a string to it so that it could be thrown out and pulled back, and this he enjoyed. At this time my interpretations were based on the idea of there being a bad, frightening mother that he wanted to be rid of; it was difficult, however, to see why he focused so much on the baby doll. I suggested that it might be the baby he feared was inside me or his mother; he did not respond much to this idea, but when I said that the baby was also the baby part of himself, he laughed and became more active.

Gradually, excursions became less frequent and concurrently he started making approaches to my body. He would pinch my hands, going on to hitting them, push my arms and head about, or hit my head. He came closer and closer until he eventually leaned up against me in an almost affectionate manner. Next he started sitting on my knee and, since it is supposed that autistic children have a defective body-image that they can be helped to form, I stroked his body and put my arms round him. He seemed to like this and it stimulated him to further attacks of the same kind, to which he now added hair-pulling, twisting my nose, shutting my mouth and then opening it. This led on to rough-and-tumble games on the couch, and ended with sitting on my knee, which became an automatic ritual; he pulled my arms round him and looked at my watch in typical autistic fashion. Yet on two occasions he gave me a hug and seemed pleased to do so, though it did not carry much feeling of affection with it. In the rough and tumble I took care that if the puzzled pained expression came into his face I at once stopped whatever I was doing.

The origin of these developments may have been a change at home. The rough-and-tumble games started when James's mother enjoyed 'romping' with him and, as his stepfather was away, she could do more of it at that time. His attacks on me could also be compared to those he sometimes made on his mother, whom he had hit quite hard several times; and once he had rushed out of his home to hit the family car with a hammer.

By now he was going to a small group in which attempts at education were begun. Not much progress was made and he began to become aggressive with the other children, which in the end led to his being excluded. As his aggression was, in a limited way, accessible to me, I decided to try and reduce his acting out. It was much easier than before and interpretations helped. These contained the idea of his wanting me to be all round him because I was good, but he feared that bad people, such as his mother sometimes turned into, were outside the room, and it was this that made him want to run outside to make sure they were not there. It was noticeable that one place he consistently looked into was the lavatory.

When in my room, which was now often for the whole interview, he brought magazines, usually *Woman's Own*. At first he seemed interested in shoes, but not consistently; also frequently in aeroplanes and motor cars and once in a Venetian blind. He cut or tore out pages on which the objects were pictured and took them away with him. He scribbled with chalks, often drawing circular whirls. Sometimes clear images were represented, and there was one like a sun, brown outside, white inside, with black lines coming out of it. The word 'the' was sometimes put in the middle. He also started obsessive drawing of coloured clocks.

I continued to interpret along the same lines of his wanting to be inside me and part of me. Once, inside the room for the whole interview, James began dividing the floor up into the parts of it that could be stepped on and those that could not, or only in a special way. The division was between the parts that were carpeted and those that were not. He jumped over the bare floor or would climb from the chair to the table or the couch without touching the floor. When he did touch the bare floor he walked on his knees. This could be compared to the permitted and forbidden parts of the house when he was not in my room, and both might be considered as his feelings about the good and bad (safe and unsafe) parts of myself.

The importance that the room had taken on was dramatically illustrated by an unfortunate incident. One day he came when it was occupied by a doctor and another child. He tried to enter the room, but I had to restrain him. He looked into the room, but I prevented him going farther. He was terrified and retreated into the secretary's office and became inaccessible. He clearly wanted to go away, would not go into the other treatment-room, and the interview ended early as his one desire seemed to be to get away. The routine of arriving exactly on time and waiting meticulously until the end, timed by my watch, had broken down altogether: he became isolated and alone. Probably this meant that the obsessional-like ritual he had been using to keep bad objects at bay was destroyed, and so the room was filled with them. The next interview was better and he wanted me to put my arms round him, for by now he enjoyed my doing so.

At this time I found that if I delayed entering the treatment-room James would push me in and shut the door. Now that he was in the treatment-room for most of the time it was easier to interpret and the patterns of his activities made more sense. It was also clear that he wanted me there and enjoyed, or rather was amused by, what I said. Also, some of his activities were like those his mother had described at home, such as dropping pencils, turning off the gas-tap, etc., so there was a clear equation between his mother and myself.

I interpreted the good and bad parts of the room as the good and bad parts of himself and his mother, both of which I myself could also feel like (this is a condensed statement). I identified the couch with his good mummy, for he did something like romping on it or danced up and down and wriggled about on it. Then he would take objects from me; once it was a match, out of my box of matches, which he put in his mouth and sucked and chewed. I interpreted this as being *his* good mummy-breast, which was like my pipe, which was *my* good mummy that I was sucking and chewing. This made him laugh, drop my matches on the floor and then go and dance about on the couch.

Besides this his ritual of sitting on my knee returned and he became more insistent about having my arms round him, and I linked this up with the circular scribbles James sometimes made. He would make them and then sit on my lap and pull my arms round him. He would insist on this by attacking them if I did not do so, pulling them upwards, twisting my hand round or pulling my little finger back until it hurt. These activities would stop if I put my arms as he wanted them. Towards the end of the interview he especially needed my left arm round him because he needed to inspect my watch and put his fingers on the hands to be sure of the time of departure.

At this time he also started to pass flatus quite frequently and this seemed related to the smell of the pipe I smoked; he would laugh and giggle about it, more so when on one occasion I did it involuntarily. He also giggled at my watch.

A number of acts took place at this time that were more communicative. Once, when he was suffering from a headache, he put my hands on each side of his head; his mother had said that he did this at home. Also I found by chance that if I stroked him up his spine he would lean forward and emit a peculiar howling noise as if he were being tortured, and that is how he looked. After it was all over he began to smile.

Another sign of James's positive feeling about me was shown by the following event. He brought into the room a large volume of Christmas cards pasted onto the leaves of the book. He selected a picture of the 'Laughing Cavalier' and, after hesitating, he looked at me, cut it out and took it away. At this time it was rare for him to look at me at all; indeed his visual avoidance was increasing. In addition, he would stay in the room with the door shut for the whole time and more than once he overstayed his time.

Visual Avoidance

This increased until most interviews became organized so that he did not look at me. He walked backwards into the room and sat on my lap looking forward into the room. As time went on I dissuaded him from sitting on me—the whole procedure having become ritualized—and I found he would accept my sitting behind him. Then he would concentrate on magazines; again *Woman's Own* or *Ideal Home* predominated and food advertisements engaged his attention most. If I moved from my position so that he might see me, he turned his head away.

This change meant that he did not inspect my watch and had to find another way of being sure of the time. There was a clock that struck the half-hours and he listened for this and then went into the secretary's room to check the time by the clock there before departing.

The visual avoidance diminished temporarily when I told James that perhaps he was afraid that I would look peculiar if he saw me stiff and upright. This I said partly because he had taken my glasses off and looked through them, and partly because a new kind of drawing had begun at home, of stiff upright shapes, which he knew his mother had brought to the clinic for me to see. As his visual avoidance diminished he would look at me and then turn away, making sucking and eating movements with his mouth. At times he would look straight at me in the way children can. As an aspect of not looking at me, he sat at a table with me behind him, looking first at the magazines and tearing some of the pictures out. Some he kept, others he threw at me over the back of his head. This increased so that he did not tear out a special picture but ripped up the magazines and threw the bits over his head. Other objects followed—pictures he had made, chalks and toys.

Besides these activities, James started using toys very much more. He took up once again some activities of the early period but in different and more vigorous ways. He ripped the clothes off little dolls with a knife and started breaking up small toys or taking them to pieces; some he took away with him. He used small clockwork toys ingeniously: most of them were put in his mouth or touched and he would wind up clockwork cars, then put the key in his mouth and let the car revolve as the spring unwound. He also put glass balls in his mouth and spit them out. He started tearing up paper with his mouth and found a large black ball that he sucked and bit. The increase in the way he used his mouth did not, however, modify the chewing of his thenar eminence when he became agitated.

A new kind of communication started at this time. James would point imperiously with his finger at an object he wanted me to fetch for him, which he could easily obtain for himself. After giving me directions several times he would get up from his chair and go and get it, being careful to keep to the safe areas of the room. This activity developed so that later on he would stamp and chew his hand if I did not do as he instructed.

Drawing and painting also became a more prominent feature of his activities, which were to develop later into 'house-decorating'. He also started using the water-pistol, squirting it into the sand-tray, on to the wall or on to my shoe, in which he was beginning to take an interest. Once he started masturbating and then his whole appearance changed and his eyes became sparkling and bright. (Upon enquiry, his mother said that he had done this at home and she had stopped him.) It may be relevant that he had once urinated on a carpet at home and this had also been stopped with characteristic firmness.

At this time James's mother telephoned several times to say that her son was ill, thus missing appointments. Eventually I encouraged her to bring him in spite of his condition. When he arrived James spent the time inert, curled up in a chair, looking pale and helpless. When I said it was time to go, he got up, went out of the room and was sick over his mother. I told him

that it was good to be sick, it got rid of all the bad stuff inside
him (thinking of all the toys crowded together behind a barrier).
Mother was pleased with this and glad that I thought his illness
emotional. James recovered quickly and there was no recurrence
of the 'illness'.

Painting now occupied him much more. He started smearing
paints on many pieces of paper, different colours separated at
first, and later one colour on top of the other. Sometimes he
painted circles and oval shapes. At this time he also developed
his oral activities. He put the water-pistol in his mouth and
squirted into it. I provided a babies' bottle and this he sucked,
chewed and twisted round in his mouth, or took the teat off
and used residual water in the bottle for mixing paints. He also
developed a new method of coming into the room: he arrived
at the door and then bent his body forward at a right angle; he
skirted round the walls laughing, but was careful not to look at
my face. He did, however, look at **my** shoes, in which (as I have
mentioned) he had been showing interest by glancing at them
and bending down to look at them; shoes had also interested
him in the magazines. Once at the table and the painting well
under way, he started making baby noises, gurgling and
becoming quite excited; then he would turn round and look
directly at me for a short time. Sometimes he would stop
smearing paint and would chalk words: THE MAR with two
marks after it; MUNNY in blue, followed by THE MUM OF MY,
followed by SUNNY with a sun on top of it, repeated with a
larger sun and smaller letters. Painting led to quite a mess on
the table which at first he always cleared up meticulously, putting objects away in a cupboard and the drawer of the table. He
began to modify this by passing objects over to me, still sitting
behind him, so that the table was clear at the end of the
interview.

The paintings and drawings of clocks in colour became a
regular feature. They always represented real clocks and
watches but there were sometimes numbers (always 1 to 12)
drawn separate from them. The times at which the hands were
placed represented real times, the start or ending times of
interviews predominating. On occasion James would occupy
himself with other objects, painting a cardboard doll's-house,
taking the objects out of a box and then making circular blobs
inside (possibly this represented taking a clock to pieces and

putting the wheels back inside—he had been interested in taking clocks to pieces at home).

Passing objects over the top of his head reached a climax when he painted the doll's-house, put his name on it, took everything out of it and handed it over to me. There was a pause and then the doll's-house furniture came over, and finally he fetched a real chair and that came over too. I told him I thought this meant giving himself to me when he felt empty, and wanting me to be with him and make a home for him so that we could be together all the time. This idea was supported by the way he was taking objects away from the clinic when he went home. After this the behaviour stopped almost entirely and I started to explore where he wanted me to be in the room. I sat beside James and asked him: he pointed in two directions—the one where I was sitting, the other in the old position; then he looked at me, covering up the left eye, nearest to me. Mostly, however, he still wanted me sitting behind him, but he would use his hand as a 'looking glass' to pretend he could see what I was doing.

The interviews now developed into cleaning-up days and messy ones. When he was not going to clear up he looked out of the window at whichever parent had brought him; they were often sitting in the car, which was in full view of the window. When he left the room tidy he did not look out, so I told him that he was sorting me out from his parents, recognizing the difference between us about messiness.

He evidently understood this for there was a considerable change. He started playing in the sand-tray; further, he took a handful of sand and put it on my lap and then wanted to pour water on as well. When I deflected him from doing this, he put it on the cushion of the other chair and put it in the wet sand-tray, from which I removed it. Next time he put the table in the sand-tray, covered it with sand and then poured water over it.

James's activities now developed. He would fill the basin with water and pull out the plug, retreat to the other end of the room and wait with excited anticipation. A climax was reached when the water started to make a noise as the basin emptied. He became very excited, jumping about and emitting 'dug-dug' noises, something like the exhaust of a diesel engine or, more probably, the Underground trains. I told him I thought he wanted to release noises inside himself like bowel noises (flatus cf. supra). He at once collected toys, put them in the cupboard, shut the door and put a chair in front of it. I told him he was afraid of the toys coming to life and pushing out like faeces. He became very quiet after this and looked out of the window. He returned, however, to the activities centring on the sink, mixed sand and water in it and then pulled out the plug. The interpretations I have detailed seemed the ones that were particularly meaningful to him, but I made others related to myself and his mother as 'lavatory mothers'.

James's feelings were closely related to looking, and one day I took this up with him as follows. He took some toy houses, painted them and laid them on one side so that the underneath could be seen: he inspected them carefully. His behaviour was dextrous and precise and this I appreciated and told him so, adding that he was also exposing the underneath parts just as sometimes he wanted to see the underneath parts of his mother, and because the toys in the room were mine he wanted also to look at me as well. He then went and picked up a small box, which he painted brown inside; he put it on the mantlepiece where I could see it. As he did so he moved and stood right in front of me so that his buttocks were a few inches in front of my face. His trousers were brown and I reflected that he was showing me how much he wanted me to look into his good brown inside and that he wanted his mother to like him that way, but she would not.

There was a small telescope among the toys; he picked this up and looked through it at the house across the road. In it were some nurses (it was a nurses' home) so I said it was they that he was looking at. Next he took the water-pistol, painted it and put it away again; then cleaned out the sand-tray, put a basin of sand in it and moved it carefully over to the window. I commented that he was letting me know that he wanted the nurse-mothers to look into his insides, which he had made good. The interview ended with a thorough tidy-up, with all the small objects, including the waste-paper basket, put in the cupboard, the door of which was shut. The chairs were then arranged round the room. He departed exactly on time.

From time to time James visited the clinic secretary's room. He would go there and sometimes use the typewriter for a short time; the secretary helped him. His interest was in the use of the machine, for there did not seem any sense in what he typed;

numbers featured in it, and occasional words. At one time he visited the room regularly before and after the sessions; he insisted on looking in the drawers of the desk, which he would also lock up, handing over the keys when he had done so only if asked for them. If the request was not made he would hide them. One day he rushed excitedly out of the secretary's room. He held a key in his hand; it unlocked the drawer of the play-room table. Some time before, when tidying up, he would put chalks and paper there, lock the drawer and put the key in the play-room cupboard. Somebody had removed it from there, but he had not seemed disturbed; now he had found the key, which had been lost months earlier. I have described this event as an example of how acute his observation could be, how tenacious his memory, and how he could work out an idea of what had happened and how to restore the lost object.

Painting activity developed in a new direction. He stopped using paper and started painting the window-frames with poster paint (his mother decorated the house at home). Then he opened the window and painted the brickwork outside it, in full view of his father or mother sitting in the car. He also 'decorated' the window-panes with names and words, so that they could be read more clearly from outside but were reversed from inside the room. He was especially fond of painting his own name and also SUSAN (ᴎAꙄUꙄ, as I saw it).

When not painting in this way, James would put the table in front of the window, lie on it and manipulate the soil in the window-box that was there; if some soil split over, he did not bother much about clearing it up. From time to time he would look over his shoulder and wriggle in an almost sexual or flirtatious way. Whether this was so or not, he looked pleased until I came very close, then he would point vigorously to the chair. I tested this sequence several times; it was always the same. Activity at the water-basin pleased him more now, and he danced and leaped about looking radiant and almost happy; when not behaving like this, he would often turn his head towards me and bite his hand, as if pleased to be doing it.

At this time I was interpreting that there was a good James and a bad one too. The bad one had worries about his parents and what they would do about the activities he was pursuing. It may have been these that made him dare to show them something of what he did with me by painting where they could see it. In reality it surprised them but they accepted it as part of treatment. Another line of interpretation focused on his oral activities and frightening wishes to bite parts of me, which made him chew himself to stop his oral attacks on me.

The Barrier

At one time James seemed almost to welcome my existence but this did not last. He started to enter the room first, shut the door and put a chair against it. I dealt with this by pushing against it from time to time, or knocking on the door, more to assure him that I was still there than with hope of entering the room. This went on for several weeks; once I pushed against the door and he was evidently not in his usual position for I was able to enter the room. I went and sat on the table where he usually sat. After a moment's hesitation, he pushed the chair against the shut door and sat in it as if I were outside. Later he turned the chair round so that he sat with his back to me, as if recognizing that I was in the room and he could not exclude me in the usual way. On other occasions I wedged the door open with my foot, which protruded into the room. It was then that this object clearly began to fascinate him for he would lean over his chair and peer at it until it went away. On another occasion I pushed into the room and then he ran away, sat on the table and drew the curtains round him so that he could not be seen. The curtain protected him.

To bypass this situation, I arranged to be in the room first. He went back to coming in bent forward so that his body was almost horizontal. It occurred to me, thinking over this behaviour, that his body was about on the level of my penis and that he could look at my shoe as he came in—this might represent my sticking-out penis. This idea gained support from remembering that he knew about the erectile behaviour of his own since he had discovered masturbation. After entering the room he regularly went and lay on the table looking out of the window.

After a short time I interpreted as follows. His bad eyes wanted to look at my penis but he was stopping them doing so by looking out of the window. This made him screw up his eyes and point vigorously out at his stepfather, who was sitting in his car in full view. I then told him he must have felt like this for a long time and that he had felt my penis was bad and black like my shoe, and he feared he would see it sticking out, because it was like his own penis that moved about and became erect, and which his mother had not liked when it wet the floor nor when he played with it.

There was no immediate response, though he stopped pointing out of the window and simply lay passive on the table. Next time, however, he was different. He spent less time in the secretary's room and went to the lavatory before coming into my room, upright and looking directly at me. He spent about one third of the interview looking at where my penis was, laughing, giggling and making pleased noises. (It was reported by his mother that, about this time, he had been annoying his father by looking at him and giggling.)

All his visual avoidance had gone and I talked about his behaviour and how it followed on from the last time we met. At one time he turned to the window and handled the earth, but only for a short time, after which he sat behind me making pleased noises. Finally he came and sat opposite me with his legs crossed and started to masturbate a little. His face was loving and contented as he put his tongue out and held it between his lips. I said that his tongue was (represented) my penis that he wanted in his mouth, as a baby had a breast. These were the essential interpretations, which I elaborated on, linking up his interest in clocks and their penis-like hands.

It was unfortunate, and perhaps disastrous, that these apparently very productive interviews took place just before my holiday. James knew about it beforehand but still to leave him after this development must have been a serious trauma.

When I came back he had reverted to his old behaviour. I repeated my interpretation. He laughed, but no change in behaviour took place. I interpreted his despair at my going away but nothing happened and it seemed the end of his trust in me. From now on he seemed to obstruct all verbal approaches by me. For some time he seemed more communicative, but this did not last. For a time he still came into the room looking away from me. He then took an armchair, turned it with its back to me, and put it close to the door by which he came into the room. He sat curled up in it for a moment, then looked over the back in my direction and screwed his eyes tightly shut, so that he could not see me if I made an interpretation; this behaviour ceased almost completely when I stopped talking. Sometimes he started making gurgling noises and if I made some too it would amuse him, but he never repeated the noises I made. As time went on James would relax, turn over to sit in the normal position or explore the door-surface with his hands, paying particular attention to the cracks or areas in which the paint-surface was defective. He sometimes made circular movements with his arms, sometimes singing tunes at the same time. Once or twice he would make excursions from his chair to look out of the window to where his father or mother could be seen in the car, or from where he could take a look at a clock. It was a quick look, after which he returned to his chair. On one occasion he came early and went into my room, which was empty. When I came in he was standing up in the corner of the room interested in some toys. There was no time to see what he was doing, for as I came in he collapsed on to the floor like lightning, doubled up, his face on the floor and his hands in front of it palms downwards. It reminded me of the way eastern people abase themselves before a god.

I came in and shut the door; he made a bolt for the chair. When I went to my own, he then arranged his in the accustomed position. He went on to sing parts of a hymn, 'Praise my soul the King of Heaven'. This suggests he was bowed down before me because I was good in an idealized sense and so not accessible and even dangerous.

There were times when he was accessible and reactive. I do not refer only to occasions when he seemed to communicate, as when he fell on the floor and then sang a tune that seemed to link up with his behaviour, but also to times when he gave up his visual avoidance and I made interpretations to which he replied in sign language—it now always negated what I said. Sometimes James would not sit in his chair by the door but would come over and sit behind me and let me look at him over the back of my chair. But I must not sit up, for then he would show rapid avoidance-reactions. If, however, I looked and talked in the right way he would respond and a loving, even doting, look would appear in his eyes and face. It would come and go, alternating with a pained, disorganized, agonized appearance—was he beginning to suffer?

Behaviour of this kind went on for several months, and then he simply came in, lay on the table and looked out of the window. It is true that there had been long periods before when nothing seemed to happen, but this time there seemed to be a greater barrier than ever before. As he had reached fifteen, the school-leaving age, beyond which child guidance treatment was not supposed to extend, I ended interviews. It was a bitter blow to his mother, who has not communicated with me since.

I understand this last period as due to my having become 'the devil's advocate', i.e., somebody whom James loved and who yet was so 'evil' that all his defences had to be mobilized against him. Had I reached the core of his autism, which I was not able to handle? In this ending period James made me depressed, inducing feelings of hopelessness and despair; these contributed to my ending the treatment. Was this like the mother's underlying depression introjected by him and then being forced into me? These are the questions that this case raised at the end, and I think that, once having started a case like this, I would not end it again on my own initiative.

Discussion

I have described in some detail a case with a depressing outcome: so many hopes were destroyed that it sometimes seemed impossible to go on. This result might have been expected and one may question whether all that work was worthwhile. I have not, however, found a detailed account by an analyst of a case like this; on the contrary, the tendency has been to describe a favourable outcome. Tustin does so in her book, and, though Bettelheim reports a poor result in 20 per cent of cases, in his case studies he records only one failure, due to parents removing a child from his orthogenic school.

It is useful to show that cases of autism can be treated psychotherapeutically, but we also want to know about failures, and the study of them is perhaps more important, just because we know that some at least benefit. I shall argue that failure was due to the intensity and nature of the barrier that exists between the child and the environment, meaning parents and their surrogates, and that this tended to induce depression in those closest to him. It is perhaps the depression that he has never reached himself, because his mother could not allow it in herself. The pattern of conflict centred on the splitting of good from bad objects, which ran right through the treatment from beginning to end. Between them there was a barrier of such strength that, though it seemed to modify itself from time to time, and so gave hope of a change, it only reasserted itself with renewed vigour at the end. Why? This question cannot be answered from the material.

Environment

James's mother corresponded closely to those described by Kanner, Rimland and Tustin. Unlike the one in Tustin's experience, she was a poor informer; indeed, throughout the treatment, she never gave more than short, though sometimes pregnant, statements about herself and James. But she was not a 'refrigerator mother', nor was she rejecting in the ordinary sense. Indeed, she put herself out to look after James, and it was not she, but I, who gave up hope. Though a controlling, obsessional character, she was rather 'hot' and, when roused, her affect would come to the surface in no uncertain manner. Further, she could drop her high standards when supported; for instance, over James's feeding behaviour. She seemed, however, unable to tolerate other sorts of mess and particularly urination. She was quite capable of appreciating James's clever tricks, even though they were at her expense, and she did not become angrily punitive, even when at one period he took off the hands of her clocks, dug up her plants etc. She was, however, firm and incisive in her disapproval. Her standards were expressed very much in terms of good and bad behaviour: James was improving if he behaved well, and not improving if he behaved badly. She seemed to have a good estimate of James's violence, and she controlled it as she controlled her own, having a mixture of anxiety and enjoyment in it.

Her physical relations with James were to treat him rather like an animal, in that she would pick him up if possible or romp with him. This was fully confirmed in James's treatment which showed that he was able to allow, manage and sometimes enjoy physical contacts, though he very seldom initiated them and eventually vigorously rejected them altogether.

Mother seemed best able to relate to her son in constructional games, like making models of houses in cardboard. She provided him with Triang toys, jigsaw puzzles, etc., and she taught him carpentry, at which she was adept.

James's stepfather expressed primitive aggression and this was sometimes directed against James, who was at first said to be terrified. As he grew up, however, he ceased to be afraid and would provoke it by stamping about, slamming doors or giggling at him. If attacked, however, James would cower down like an animal but soon recover. Stepfather was said to be fond of James and he co-operated meticulously in bringing him to and from the clinic. I believe this description of James's reaction to his father's rage to be correct, for at one time I tried being angry with James and he behaved as described. It did not interfere noticeably with my relation to him afterwards.

It would be quite wrong to say there was no relation between James and his mother; indeed, in many ways the two were exceptionally close. She seemed to, as it were, surround him and be part of him on all sides. This was reflected in the treatment, and one could even parallel her affective uncommunicativeness with his. She hardly seemed to have many words to express her feelings, perhaps because of their strength.

What were the activities James could engage in that mother would not tolerate? Running off round the building? He would run or wander off and go into other people's houses. Hide and seek? It is true that she made no mention of these games, but he would play tricks on her of a hide-and-seek kind and this annoyed her, although she appreciated their ingenuity. Painting, drawing, cutting-out or extracting pages from magazines were all home activities. When they became compulsively ritualized I asked him to stop and he did so. It may here be relevant to remark, that he did many things, like helping his mother to tidy up, wash up, lay the table, that she appreciated. Throwing objects out of the window, destroying toys, masturbating all took place at home and were firmly stopped. James did not persist. We are left with a range of activity associated with making more serious mess in the sand-tray, all sexual acts and feelings, and all those activities that established a barrier between us, shutting doors, turning his back or ending up with persistent and implacable rejection —total rejection of everything I said for long periods and especially at the end, and no activity that I could interpret.

The features of the interviews that were different from home were my greater tolerance of home behaviour because the situation was different so that I did not need to interfere much.

It may seem that I did interfere at crucial points i.e. over the 'house-painting' and objecting to mess that was directed at me and that I missed opportunities that would have led to breaking down his obsessional behaviour; but acting out had only led to another obsession.

Because other therapists had noticed this with their cases, I stopped the activity because verbalizing its content seemed more desirable. This may have been wrong, for Bettelheim suggests that there can be a need for regression to take place in which the child becomes incontinent once more, and relearns control in his own way rather than his mother's. If, however, his mother is to be believed, toilet-training was skilful and not over-organized. It is just possible that his mother might have collaborated over such a regression had James acted out at home. Mother could have allowed him to become grubby and this might have been built on.

She handled the situation over the food, which was somewhat like an infant's use of faeces, but James did not act at home over his excrement in a way that his mother could get help over. Much more aggression by James would have been needed, much more determination in this field than he was capable of. The most likely construction is, however, that both mother and child were much too frightened of their anal aggression so that they colluded in making the reliving of anal feeling impossible, even though James received help over it from me. But if this line were taken on other cases with obsessional parents, much analytic therapy would not take place, and so it might have been expected that by more skilled interpretation and use of the transference such a collusion might be resolved without acting out at home. That this could not be done with James suggests three lines of thought.

1. He was not being seen often enough—twice a week only is little for such a severe case.

2. It could not be done in the home environment. This does not seem justified though Bettelheim always treated his patients away from home so as to take the child away from the malign influence of the mother.

3. There was a great deal of acting out that I played in with. It is true that after two years I decided to stop it, but it could have left a good memory, which enhanced the feeling of my now being an enemy who had stopped colluding with his defence

systems, and was consequently against them and a traitor. Also it may have enhanced his tendency to act rather than translate actions into words. The idea behind my collusion was to try entering into James's world as far as possible and lure him out of it. I do not think this was successful. As part of this idea, combined with the notion that James's body-image could be improved, from time to time, and over most of the treatment span, I allowed and fostered physical contact. I am doubtful of its value.

Though no two cases are strictly comparable, the cases in which I did not actively do this were more satisfactory: they talked and became less autistic than James. Furthermore, if the idea is to attempt reliving infantile traumata, then why not let the child's mother do it herself? In another case (John) that I treated this happened. The mother allowed extensive use of her body. She arranged her home largely for his benefit. There were no breakable objects in the rooms, which were none the less comfortable, and the child could run around without being anxious lest he should break objects that he sometimes threw on the floor. His oral sadism was also very marked and took the form of chewing up blankets that his mother left on his bed for him to use. In this case my activity was confined to interpretation, though sometimes I acted out according to John's directions. He developed a clearly defined obsessional neurosis, matching closely that of his father, from whom his mother separated when her child was three years old.

But there is a problem about how to talk to a non-talking child. This subject is made easier with those children who verbalize some of their responses to therapeutic interventions; James did not but only gave more or less clear indications that he had understood and valued them. Sometimes there were small changes in the way he behaved, sometimes clear ones; twice they were dramatic. If, however, I compare what I said with the more subtle communications developed by Tustin, it is clear that I was mostly interpreting in areas that did not lead in the direction she holds to be central: they did not reach out to the infant depression that she postulates as basic to autism.

In part this may have been due to James's having entered the latency period, but there were a number of behaviour patterns on which she lays stress that might have been more subtly taken up. There was enough to indicate similarities with her case material—the mother all round him and his rejection of her (mummy gone, in the throwing away of objects): there were also the swirling patterns in his drawings and wrapping himself round in the curtain, and being wrapped round in my arms and the 'dark hole', i.e., dark room. These I interpreted in a way close to hers.

I therefore think that, though a good deal of refinement of interpretation could now be made, and this would have made a difference, there is no evidence that more subtle communications would have been decisive.

There remains the original trauma, the combination of love, fear and implacable denial. It was the last that took over but before it I obtained a glimpse of the terrible and pathetic quandary in which James was placed. It was as if there was a powerful element that could not allow love to mature—it was too dangerous.

It may be thought that it was the arrival at adolescence that was determinative, and that I was not observing the original autism. This would be too simple. Without doubt his sexual impulses had to be warded off, and a regression took place; projective identifications increased, and other early infantile patterns were revived.

My conclusion is that the barrier systems that James showed were not so much defence-systems of the ego but the primary defence-systems of the self, which had persisted from his infancy and become organized into obsessional structures.

It is from the detailed investigation of cases like James that we may hope to arrive at greater understanding of the condition as a whole, by arriving at general propositions. A feature of James's behaviour that I want to comment on further is the bits of behaviour that were not autistic; indeed, one might call them, if not normal, at least approximating to health. There was his capacity to relate to me in games of hide-and-seek, and there was his capacity to understand quite complex ideas and to devise even witty reactions to his mother's requests.

It is on these positive capacities that any analytic attempt must rely; that I did so must be apparent, that they could not help James sufficiently is to be regretted. It is, however, relevant to observe that it was possible to draw out the normal parts of James, and it is thought that a great deal can be done by using methods similar to the ones I employed: they are all educative, whether the method be to engage in establishing physical contact, or to use special educational methods. My observations indicate the likely reason for their partial success and also why they cannot hope to be therapeutic of autism: they relate to the relatively normal parts of the child and leave the essential disorder uninfluenced. It is a negative conclusion again, but it is in line with those of therapists like Bettelheim, who hold that the best hope of benefit to autistic children is to work out ways in which the environment can allow deintegration to take place, and meet the child's approach when it appears. To provoke relationship is to prevent access to the autistic core, which pervades all but a tiny part of the child's ego.

BIBLIOGRAPHY

ALDRIDGE, M. (1959). 'The birth of the black and white twins.' *J. analyt. Psychol.*, **4**, 1.

ANTONY, J. (1958). 'An experimental approach to the psychopathology of childhood autism.' *Brit. J. med. Psychol.*, **31**, 3.

BALINT, M. (1968). *The basic fault*. London, Tavistock.

BENDER, L. (1953). 'Childhood schizophrenia.' *Psychiat. Quart.*, **27**.

BETTELHEIM, B. (1967). *The empty fortress*. New York, Free Press; London, Collier-Macmillan.

BETZ, B. (1947). 'Study of tactics for resolving the autistic barrier in the psychotherapy of the schizophrenic barrier.' *Am. J. Psychiat.*, **104**.

BION, W. R. (1955). 'Language of the schizophrenic.' In *New directions in psychoanalysis*. London, Tavistock.

BOWLBY, J. (1969). *Attachment and loss*. I. London, Hogarth.

BRADLEY, C. (1941). *Schizophrenia in childhood*. New York, Macmillan.

CAHEN, R. (1955). 'Psychotherapie de C. G. Jung.' In *Encyclopédie Medico-Chirurgicale*. Paris.

CALL, J. D. (1964). 'Newborn approach behaviour and early ego development.' *Int. J. Psycho-Anal.*, **45**, 23.

COLMAN, R. W., KRIS, E. & PROVENCE, S. (1953). 'Variations in early parental attitudes.' In *The psychoanalytic study of the child.*, **8**. New York Int. Univ. Press; London, Hogarth.

DIATKINE, R. (1960). 'Reflections on the genesis of psychotic object relations in the young child.' *Int. J. Psycho-Anal.*, **41**, 4–5.

FORDHAM, F. 'Ruthless greed'. Unpublished.

——(1963). 'Myths, archetypes and patterns of childhood.' *Harvest*, **9**.

FORDHAM, M. (1944). *The life of childhood*. London, Routledge and Kegan Paul.
——(1947). 'Integration, disintegration and early ego development.' *Nervous child*, **6**, 3.
——(1952). 'A child guidance approach to marriage.' In *New developments in analytical psychology*. London, Routledge, 1957.
——(1957). 'Biological theory and the concept of archetypes.' Ibid.
——(1957a). 'Reflections on image and symbol.' Ibid.
——(1957b). 'The origins of the ego in childhood.' Ibid.
——(1957c). 'Some observations on the self and the ego in childhood.' Ibid.
——(1957d). 'Child analysis.' Ibid.
——(1958). 'Individuation and ego development.' *J. analyt. Psychol.* **3**, 2.
——(1960). 'The emergence of a symbol in a five-year-old child.' Chap. 10 in *Children as individuals*. London, Hodder & Stoughton 1969.
——(1960a). 'Counter transference.' In *Analytical psychology: a modern science*. London, Heinemann. 1973.
——(1963). 'The empirical foundation and theories of the self in Jung's works.' Ibid.
——(1969). *Children as individuals*. London, Hodder and Stoughton.
FREUD, A. (1960). Discussion of Dr. John Bowlby's paper: 'Grief and mourning in infancy and early childhood'. In *The psychoanalytic study of the child.*, **15**. New York, Int. Univ. Press; London, Hogarth.
FREUD, S. (1900). 'The interpretation of dreams.' *Standard edition.*, **4 & 5**. London, Hogarth.
——(1914). 'On narcissism: an introduction'. Ibid, **14**.
——(1916—17). 'Introductory lectures on psychoanalysis.' Ibid, **16**.
——(1920). 'Beyond the pleasure principle.' Ibid, **18**.
——(1923). 'The ego and the id.' Ibid, **19**.
——(1924). 'The economic problem of masochism.' Ibid, **19**.
——(1937). 'Analysis terminable and interminable.' Ibid, **23**.
——(1940). 'An outline of psychoanalysis.' Ibid. **23**.
FÜRST, EMMA. (1909). 'Statistical investigations on word-association and on familial agreement in reaction type amongst uneducated persons.' In *Studies in word association*. Ed. C. G. Jung. Trans Eder. London, Routledge. 1969.

GELEERD, E. R. (1949). 'The psychoanalysis of a psychotic child.' In *The psychoanalytic study of the child* **3–4**. New York, Int. Univ. Press.
GELEERD, R. G. (1963). 'Evaluation of Melanie Klein's *Narrative of a child analysis*.' *Int. J. Psycho-Anal.*, **44**, 4.
GOLDFARB, W. (1961). Childhood schizophrenia. Cambridge, Mass., Harvard University Press.
GLOVER, E. (1943). 'The concept of dissociation'. In *On the early development of the mind*. London, Imago 1956.
GORDON, R. (1961). 'The death instinct and its relation to the self.' *J. analyt. Psychol.* **6**, 2.

HARTMANN, H. (1950). 'Comments on the psychoanalytic theory of the ego.' In *The psychoanalytic study of the child.*, **5**. New York, Int. Univ. Press; London, Hogarth.

The self and autism

HAWKEY, L. (1945). 'Play analysis: case study of a nine-year-old child.' *Brit. J. med. Psychol.* **20**, 3.
——(1947). 'The witch and the bogey.' *Brit. J. med. Psychol.*, **20**, 3.
HEIMANN, P. (1950). 'On counter-transference.' *Int. J. Psycho-Anal.*, **31**, 1.
——(1955). 'A contribution to the re-evaluation of the Oedipus complex.' In *New directions in psychoanalysis*. London, Tavistock.
HOBSON, R. (1961). 'The archetypes of the collective unconscious.' In *Analytical psychology: a modern science*. London, Heinemann. 1973.

ISAACS, S. (1948). 'An acute psychotic anxiety occurring in a boy of four years.' In *Childhood and after*. London, Routledge and Kegan Paul.

JACOBI, J. (1953). 'Ich und Selbst in der Kinderzeichnung.' *Schweitz. Z. Psychol. anwend.* **12**, 1.
——(1967). *The way of individuation*. London, Hodder and Stoughton.
JACOBSON, E. (1964). *The self and the object world*. New York, Int. Univ. Press; London, Hogarth.
JUNG, C. G. (1909). 'The significance of the father in the destiny of the individual' in the Jahrbuch für psychoanalytische und psychopathologische Forschungen, Leipzig, **I**.
——(1910). 'Psychic conflicts in a child.' In *The Collected works of C. G. Jung.* **17**. Princeton, P.U.P., London, Routledge.
——(1913). 'The theory of psychoanalysis.' Ibid. **4**.
——(1921). *Psychological types*. Ibid. **6**.
——(1926). 'Analytical psychology and education.' Ibid. **17**.
——(1928). 'Child development and education.' Ibid. **17**.
——(1941). 'The psychological aspects of the Kore.' Ibid., **9**, 1.
——(1944). *Psychology and alchemy*. Ibid., **12**.
——(1946). 'Psychology of the transference'. Ibid. **16**.
——(1948). 'On psychic energy.' Ibid., **8**.
——(1949). 'The significance of the father in the destiny of the individual.' Ibid. **3**.
——(1951). 'Psychology of the child archetype.' Ibid. **9**.
——(1951a). *Aion*. Ibid. **9**, 2.
——(1952). *Symbols of transformation*. Ibid. **5**.
——(1963). *Memories, dreams, reflections*. London, Collins and Routledge.

KANNER, L. (1948). *Child psychiatry*. Oxford, Blackwell.
KALFF, M. D. (1962) 'Archetypus als heilender factor.' In *The archetype*. Basel/New York, Klarger.
KELLOGG, R. (1969). *Analysing children's art*. Palo Alto, National Press Books.
KLEIN, M. (1930). 'The importance of symbol-formation in the development of the ego.' In *Contributions to psychoanalysis*. London, Hogarth.
——(1932). *The psychoanalysis of children*. London, Hogarth.
——(1946). 'Notes on some schizoid mechanisms.' In *New developments in psychoanalysis*. 1952. London, Tavistock.

LEWIS, E. (1953). 'The function of group play during middle childhood in developing the ego complex.' *Brit. J. med. Psychol.*, **27**, 1/2.

Bibliography

MacDougall, J. & Leborici, S. (1969). *Dialogue with Sammy*. London, Hogarth.

Mahler, M. (1969). *On human symbiosis and the vicissitudes of individuation*. London, Hogarth.

Mahler, M. & Gosliner, R. J. (1955). 'On symbiotic child psychosis.' In *The psychoanalytic study of the child*. **10**. New York, Int. Univ. Press; London, Hogarth.

Moody, R. (1955). 'On the function of counter-transference.' *J. analyt. Psychol*. **1**, 1.

——(1961). 'A contribution to the psychology of the mother–child relationship.' In *Current trends in analytical psychology*. Ed. G. Adler. London, Tavistock.

Newton, K. (1965). 'Mediation of the image of infant–mother togetherness.' In *Analytical psychology: a modern science*. Library of Analytical Psychology. Vol. I. London, Heinemann. 1973.

Perry, J. W. (1962). 'Reconstructive process in the psychotherapy of the self'. In *Ann. N.Y. Acad*. **96**. New York.

Piaget, J. (1951). *Play, dreams and imitation in childhood*. London & Toronto, Heinemann.

Polanyi, M. (1969). *Knowing and being*. London, Routledge.

Pollock, G. M. (1964). 'On symbiosis and symbiotic neurosis.' *Int. J. Psycho-Anal*., **45**, 1.

Racker, De G. T. (1961). 'On the formulation of an interpretation.' *Int. J. Psycho-Anal*. **42**, 1–2.

Rimland, B. (1965). *Infantile autism*. London, Methuen.

Robinson, R. J. (Ed.) (1969). *Brain and early behaviour development in the foetus and baby*. London/New York, Academic Press.

Rodrigué, E. (1955). 'The analysis of a three-year-old mute schizophrenic.' In *New directions in psychoanalysis*. London, Tavistock.

Rosenfeld, H. (1965). *Psychotic states, a psychoanalytic approach*. London, Hogarth.

Searles, H. F. (1965). 'Transference psychosis in psychotherapy.' In *Collected papers*. London, Hogarth.

Sechehaye, M. H. (1951). *Symbolic realization*. New York, Int. Univ. Press.

Segal, H. (1957). 'Notes on symbol formation.' *Int. J. Psycho-Anal*. **38**, 6.

——(1964). *Introduction to the work of Melanie Klein*. London, Heinemann.

Spitz, R. (1960). 'Discussion of Dr. John Bowlby's paper "Grief and mourning in infancy and early childhood." ' In *The psychoanalytic study of the child*. **15**. New York, Int. Univ. Press.

Spitz, R. A. (1957). *No and yes*. New York, Int. Univ. Press.

Stein, L. (1967). 'Introducing not-self.' *J. analyt. Psychol*. **12**, 2.

Strachey, J. (1961). Appendix B 'The great reservoir of libido' to S. Freud: 'The ego and the id'. In *Standard edition*, **19**.

Tate, D. (1958). 'On ego development.' *J. analyt. Psychol*., **3**, 1.

——(1961). 'Invasion and separation.' *J. analyt. Psychol*., **6**, 1.

The self and autism

TEILHARD DE CHARDIN, P. (1959). *The phenomenon man.* London, Collins.
TINBERGEN, N. (1951). *The study of instinct.* London, O.U.P.
TUSTIN, F. (1972). *Autism and childhood psychosis.* London, Hogarth.

WEILAND, H. & RUDNIK, R. (1961). 'Considerations of the development and treatment of autistic child psychosis.' In *The psychoanalytic study of the child.* New York, Int. Univ. Press.
WICKES, F. E. (1966). *The inner world of childhood.* New York, Appleton.
WILLIAMS, M. (1964). 'The indivisibility of the personal and collective unconscious.' In *The archetype.* Basel and New York, Klarger.
WINNICOTT, D. W. (1952). 'Psychoses and child care.' In *Collected papers.* London, Tavistock, 1958.
——(1955). 'A case managed at home.' In *Collected papers.* London, Tavistock, 1958.
——(1965). 'A clinical study of the effect of a failure of the average expectable environment on a child's natural functioning.' *Int. J. Psycho-Anal.,* **46**, 1.
——(1965a). *The maturation process and the facilitating environment.* London, Hogarth.
——(1971). *Therapeutic consultations.* London, Hogarth.
——(1971a). *Playing and reality.* London, Tavistock.

ZUBLIN, W. (1961). 'The mother figure in the fantasies of a boy suffering from early deprivations.' In *Current trends in analytical psychology.* London, Tavistock.

Index